TEACHING CONTEMPORARY YOGA

Teaching Contemporary Yoga provides a novel look at how modern yoga is understood, practiced, and taught globally. Utilising perspectives from several academic disciplines, the authors offer an analysis of the current state of modern yoga and the possibilities for future experimentation and innovation. The authors draw on anthropological, performance, and embodiment theories to understand yoga practice as a potentially powerful ritual of transformation as well as a cultural product steeped in the process of meaning making. They craft a unique analysis that contrasts *asana* with the largely unexamined philosophy underlying the practice of *vinyasa*, while imagining a vibrant future for the evolution of yoga through excellence in teaching.

Unlike other writings about yoga, the authors offer a critique of the current practice of yoga as both diminished and utilitarian, while providing a path to reinvigorating the discipline based on current scientific knowledge and methods for teaching and practice. Along with these theoretical perspectives and the analysis of contemporary yoga in the West, the authors offer practical applications to address the challenges of teaching yoga in a society where individualism and materialism are core values. Open-ended exercises in reflection and experimentation offer opportunities for readers to apply what they have learned to their teaching and personal practice. This is a vital guide for any yoga-oriented scholar, teacher, or practitioner and is an essential companion for contemporary teacher training.

Edward Clark is the creator and artistic director of Tripsichore Yoga Theatre in London. He is internationally recognised as a teacher of advanced yoga technique and philosophy.

Laurie A. Greene, PhD, is Associate Professor of Anthropology at Stockton University and the owner of Yoga Nine studios in New Jersey. She works in clinical settings and has published numerous articles on yoga therapy.

TEACHING CONTEMPORARY YOGA

PHYSICAL PHILOSOPHY AND CRITICAL ISSUES

EDWARD CLARK AND LAURIE A. GREENE

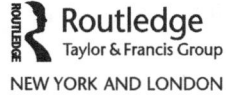

Routledge
Taylor & Francis Group

NEW YORK AND LONDON

Cover credit: Photo by Paul Dempsey, "Equillibrium"

First published 2022
by Routledge
605 Third Avenue, New York, NY 10158

and by Routledge
4 Park Square, Milton Park, Abingdon, Oxon, OX14 4RN

Routledge is an imprint of the Taylor & Francis Group, an informa business

Library of Congress Cataloging-in-Publication Data
Names: Clark, Edward (Yoga teacher), author. | Greene, Laurie A., author.
Title: Teaching contemporary yoga : physical philosophy and
critical issues / Edward Clark, Tripsichore Yoga, Laurie A. Greene,
Stockton University & Yoga Nine Studios.
Description: New York, NY : Routledge, 2022. |
Includes bibliographical references and index. |
Identifiers: LCCN 2021042377 (print) | LCCN 2021042378 (ebook) |
ISBN 9781032018775 (hardback) | ISBN 9781032018768 (paperback) |
ISBN 9781003181910 (ebook)
Subjects: LCSH: Hatha yoga–Study and teaching.
Classification: LCC RA781.7 C5786 2022 (print) |
LCC RA781.7 (ebook) | DDC 613.7/046–dc23
LC record available at https://lccn.loc.gov/2021042377
LC ebook record available at https://lccn.loc.gov/2021042378

ISBN: 9781032018775 (hbk)
ISBN: 9781032018768 (pbk)
ISBN: 9781003181910 (ebk)

DOI: 10.4324/9781003181910

Typeset in Galliard
by Newgen Publishing UK

CONTENTS

Figures

PREFACE: NOTES ON THE PROBLEM OF TRANSLATION

There are many challenges to writing a book on a complex and heterogenous tradition like yoga. The definition of yoga has and continues to be contested in both Eastern and Western contexts. Though Hindu culture has laid claims to its birth, the most recent analysis by scholars of Sanskrit suggests that the earliest physical practices (*hatha yoga*) may originate in Buddhism, as they are found in Buddhist texts (Mallinson 2019). Claims of cultural appropriation are not new to yoga, as organisations like HAF (Hindu American Foundation 2020) and others are opposed to Westerners calling what they do "yoga", and through their "Take Back Yoga" campaign have claimed that every style of yoga has, at its root, Hindu religious traditions. Most scholars of yoga convincingly argue that yoga is not a religion but a philosophical tradition that seeks spiritual ends, and that it has been and continues to be practiced in this context and outside of many religious traditions. In writing this book, we were sensitive to these claims, but agree as Andrea Jain has shown in her book, *Selling Yoga*, that, "yoga is a complex cultural product," and that it has been "continually context-sensitive, so there is no 'legitimate,' 'authentic,' 'true,' or 'original,' tradition, only contextualised ideas and practices organised around the term yoga" (2015, xvi). What we are describing here is a manifestation of the somatic practice of yoga as it is taught in mostly Western contexts.

Yoga philosophy is also complex and has a multidirectional historical trajectory. There is no clear line of philosophical development, but instead it is the result of a variety of competing traditions, many of which are poorly understood. Philosophical conjecture and practice undoubtably began in preliterate times, and texts are often obtuse in that they are steeped with metaphor or composed of coded aphorisms that are highly interpretable. A variety of texts note the wisdom of ancient teachers whose theories and practices have already been interpreted by their students.[1]

Language doesn't live on a page; it conveys meaning through the complex communications of its speakers. Writing is a convention that is devised to record language through symbols. Archaeologists are all too familiar with the limitations of using written language as a reliable record of cultural history. Ancient writing systems, in particular, have been shown to have intentionally restrictive functions (for example liturgy). Ancient Sanskrit requires both translation and interpretation, as scholars try to piece together meaning in modern times. Sanskrit is a living language,[2] and translators are well aware that language, as a living entity, is always changing and, in addition, meaning is multivariate and subject to context. We have chosen here to use Sanskrit terms as we interpret them based on a modern sensibility informed by our own yoga practices and the translations of others. In many cases, these interpretations are definitions based on popular usage. *Asana*, for example, is literally translated as "stable seat" by most philologists of Sanskrit, but it is popularly used to mean "posture" in the context of modern yoga practice. Likewise, philosophical concepts like *purusha* and *prakriti*, described by the philosopher Kapila, are denoted by words like *consciousness*, without certain knowledge of how consciousness may have been understood at the time.[3] Respecting these traditions, we have chosen to further interpret and define these terms in ways that are in accordance with a modern understanding and as part of a philosophical construct that is feasible in a Western context. This is in no way meant to disengage the Eastern origins of these philosophies, and these origins are noted.

We have attempted in this book to take a novel look at teaching yoga from a perspective that is largely influenced by aesthetic philosophy. To do so, we have made a number of choices that might initially appear perplexing. There are so many subtleties to yoga that make an all-encompassing, yet detailed, overview daunting – especially when opinions are staunchly held as to the authenticity of individual paths. In contemporary physical practice, though, there are two clearly distinct positions – neither of which seems for all intents and purposes to practically exist without the other. Throughout this book we refer to them as *vinyasa* and *asana*.

Though the literal translation of *vinyasa* is noted as "to place in a special way", vernacular use of the term has come to mean a style of practice that is based on continuous movement, guided by breath. We contrast this with *asana* practice, which, for the purposes of this book, we describe as something that is predicated on desire to achieve physical (and mental) stillness. This is colloquially practiced in the holding of postures for some effect, as is described in the hatha yoga texts.[4] When someone says, "I am practicing *asana*," they generally mean, "I am practicing postures, not the movement from posture to posture." In contrast, when a practitioner says, "I am practicing *vinyasa*," they are undoubtedly referring to a moving practice. We feel that both share methods of practice based on the possibility of experiencing something that is ineffable and aesthetically rich. In defining beauty as an experience that is uniquely felt and construed by each individual and not as the object of appreciation, we hope to shed some light on the means by which this ineffable aesthetic emotion can be cultivated through the practise of yoga and parallel it with something that can be seen in the many forms of "authentic" yoga – a knowledge of self and reality.

The naming of postures also raises vexing problems for clarity. Names attributed in either Sanskrit or English vary between orthodoxies and between individual practitioners. Since this book is written in English, describing most postures in this way provides a clarity that, in many cases, Sanskrit cannot or where a Sanskrit term is absent. Except in a few cases therefore, we use English descriptions to designate postures. Certain claims made by ancient yogis – the acquisition of powers (*siddhis*), the ability to levitate or cure all diseases, or the codification of the "subtle body" – test modern sensibilities and demonstrable scientific knowledge. We have chosen to interpret these phenomena as "metaphorical" since they would otherwise require an abandonment of the scientific worldview. For example, when engaging the body and lifting up through the centre and the spine, a practitioner might feel a sense of "lightness"; perhaps this is what the ancient yogis meant by "levitation". In an effort to be in line with scientific and Western cultural worldviews, we have also chosen to view and define concepts like subtle anatomy (*koshas, chakras, nadis*) metaphorically, rather than literally. This is not to suggest that the techniques to manipulate this energetic body are less potent, but simply imaginative rather than demonstrable. *Pratyahara, dharana,* and *dhyana* are, therefore, reinterpreted to be better understood in Western contexts that seek to integrate the imaginative and the demonstrable. In sum, the reinterpretation of these philosophical tenets and the practice of yoga described here has a long historical development in Indian culture, and a much shorter and less rooted one in the West. Our analysis recognises this truth and proposes a continuation of this rich philosophical dialogue in light of modern scientific and cultural realities.

The use of Sanskrit terms in their English translations and the contention that these definitions are fixed belies the reality of their internal variability within Sanskrit and their subsequent interpretation when translated into English. Language is symbolic – a representation of ideas – and writing is a record of language use that later enables interpretation. The use of terms in a static way serves only to disengage them from the richness of their source, for it privileges historicity over evolution of ideas.

Notes

1   *Sutras* (threads or strings) are incomplete sentences, a shorthand for a sage's teachings. These are meant to be interpreted through a guru to their students. The ambiguity of the textual rendering is intentional. Each original volume is known by its interpreter (e.g., The *Yoga Sutra* attributed to Patanjali, The *Hatha Yoga Pradipika* attributed to Svātmārāma, the *Acharyas'* – most notably Shankaracharya's – interpretation of the *Mahabharata*, et al.).

2   A living language is one that is spoken by a social group. In use, meaning is negotiated and influenced by other languages with which the social group interacts. Telugu, for example, has influenced the Sanskrit spoken in southern India. Languages inevitably change over time, despite attempts to codify and restrict them. Jamal Jones, personal communication 19 October, 2020.

3   The ambiguous nature of "consciousness" gives rise to many interpretations. Is *Purusha* "soul," "spirit," "individual," "man, the knower," etc.? *Prakriti* has a similar ambiguity, since it is defined as "nature" or "matter," and *Mulaprakriti* as "primordial," "basic," or "original" – while still meaning "that which exists in nature." (Sinha, 1986: 29).

4   *Hatha Yoga Pradipika, Gheranda Samhita, Siva Samhita,* et al.

References

Hindu American Foundation (HAF) website. Accessed 10 December, 2020. www. hinduamerican.org/projects/hindu-roots-of-yoga

Jain, Andrea. *Selling yoga: from counterculture to pop culture.* Oxford: Oxford University Press, 2015.

Mallinson, James. "The Tantric Buddhist roots of Hatha Yoga." *Advaya.* Accessed 19 April, 2019. https://advaya.co/read/2019/04/19/the-tantric-buddhist-roots-of-hatha-yoga

Sinha, Phulgenda. *The Gita as it was: rediscovering the original Bhagavad Gita.* La Salle: Open Court, 1986.

ACKNOWLEDGEMENTS

Many people have contributed to the creation of this book. We are particularly appreciative to those who read and commented upon the early drafts. Reading unfinished versions of a book is time consuming and is not an obviously gratifying activity. Some of the following people showed the extraordinary kindness of strangers, while others the patience of enduring friendship: Martin McDougall, Joseph Alter, Sarah Strauss, Anya Foxen, David Life, Ana Forrest, Erich Schiffmann, Jamal Jones, Hunter Dudkiewicz, Yenny Christine, and Andrew Eppler. Their comments and contributions were invaluable.

It is a truism of teaching that you learn from your students. The reexamination of basic premises happens, ideally, on a regular basis – sometimes instigated by dissenting opinion. This forces one to review material that has seemed so obvious it should not need explication or reconsideration. We are grateful to the students who have attended classes over the years both as enthusiastic experimenters (with what we have taught) and those who were dubious enough to provoke us to clarify our ideas. Gratitude should, of course, also be extended to our own teachers who gave us the latitude to experiment and who, through criticism and encouragement, helped us to form and begin to articulate our ideas about yoga in our own way.

A further debt is owed to various colleagues who have contributed to the formation and pursuit of ideas we have articulated: Elizabeth Connally, Nikki Durrant, Giris Rabinovitch, various Tripsichore performers and producers past and present, and all of those who we have trained as teachers – who have gone on to create their own interpretations of teaching, philosophy, and practice.

We also wish to acknowledge Sharon Garland who made the illustrations for the book and Paul Dempsey, photographer extraordinaire and friend. We are very indebted to our publisher, Anna Moore, who decided to take a chance with the manuscript, and the staff of *Routledge* for all their help in bringing this book to publication. Last, we would like to thank our parents, Jim and Katie Clark, and Marlyn and Irwin Greene, for unwavering support of our unusual and sometimes challenging interests and life choices.

Glossary of Sanskrit Terms[1]: (Literal Translations)[2]

Asana	"sitting", "seat", "posture"
Brahman	sacred utterance, absolute / eternal reality
Dharana	"supporting", "bearing", "concentration or focus"
Dhyana	"meditation", "reflection", "visualisation / imagination"
Ekagrata	"(lit.) single-pointedness", "single-mindedness", "focus"
Karma	"action (esp. of a ritual kind)", "the effect of an action", "an object of action"
Maya	"illusion", "magic," "enchantment"
Mula	"root", "source", "foundation", "origin", "cause"
Nirvana	"(lit.) to blow out", "extinguishing / extinction", "cessation", "perfect calm / happiness / bliss"
Prakriti	"creation or creativity", "nature"
Prana	"wind", "breath", "life-force"
Pranayama	"breath-restriction", "breath-control"
Pratayahara	"withdrawal", "(re-)absorption", "compression"
Purusha	"man", "person", "being", "soul"
Samadhi	"completion or accomplishment", "intense or ultimate contemplation", "final resting placing (or tomb)"
Savasana	"seated like a corpse, as if dead"

Uddiyana	"upward lifting" [position of three fingers below the navel]
Ujjayi	"conquering, victorious"
Vinyasa	"placing down", "arranging"
Yoga	"yoking", "joining", "connecting / connection", "practice or application", "effort", "magic"

NOTES

1   Within each chapter, Sanskrit terms that have been interpreted for this book are indicated in italics.
2   Jamal Jones, p.c. 21 October, 2020.

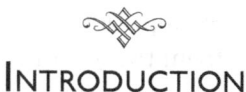

Introduction

CRITICAL ACCEPTANCE

In writing a book on teaching, as in writing any book with practical application, a number of decisions must be made. In this case, the decisions were wrought from beliefs about what best practice in teaching yoga, or teaching any discipline, entails. There are certainly basic "rules" for teaching postural yoga, as there exist underlying anatomical and functional concepts that should be followed, but these rules can be presented in a number of ways. Many texts on teaching yoga present these rules as prescriptions: "how to"s that, when followed verbatim, guarantee the path to success, but this text has other concerns. It presents instead of *prescriptive* instruction a *descriptive* one; one that asks the student, and the student of teaching, to understand underlying principles and follow them in their own way; a way that results from personal inquiry and experimentation. This theoretical perspective, called *critical acceptance*, is simply a reworking of the habit of mind known as critical thinking. It asks that one accept a hypothesis only so that it might be tested, and that, from this testing, the experimenter is able to change their mind; either maintaining the working hypothesis, modifying it, or throwing it away as the results demand.

DOI: 10.4324/9781003181910-1

1

Thinking critically is one of the most discriminating skills one can acquire. Critical thinking can be defined as the active, persistent, and careful consideration of knowledge (facts and opinions) (Dewey 1933, 118). It is a way of reflecting on one's beliefs and the reasons for them. It is a way to learn how to be persuasive and articulate, but also how to evaluate information that is commonly left unquestioned. In any discussion, one considers the purpose of the argument, the question(s) that are being posed, the assumptions that underlie the argument, the conclusions that are drawn from the argument, and the consequences of these conclusions. When one presents a position, they must make sure to state their perspective fully and clearly, elaborate on important points by expanding one's position and clarifying points when needed, and illustrating points that exemplify one's position.

Without critical thinking and discussion, a teacher's hypotheses as well as the theories of any scholar, saint, or teacher, no matter how famous, are simply *opinions*. Persuasion comes when an argument is understood (What is it?), explained (Why is it so?), and illustrated (How is it done?). Though opinions and feelings are important, in meaningful discourse they must be supported, and the teacher models this behaviour for their students to push them to practice critical acceptance as well: "listen to my theory, entertain it and test it, see what arises for you. Take notes, explore, trust the process, not me." When practiced (for critical acceptance is, above all, a practice), teachers have answers for students' queries that deny tautologies like, "because that is the sequence," or "because it is always taught that way," or "because guruji said...". Through exploration and experimentation, teachers build their own theory, based on the critical exploration of *their* teachers' hypotheses. They accept, reject, or more likely modify theory as the result of their continuing quest for answers. When a problem has not been resolved, they frankly acknowledge this to *their* students and focus their own practice on further exploration. Through the process of *deductive* reasoning, hypotheses are explored and tested. In yoga, *inductive* reasoning is equally important as a source of knowledge. Here practitioners allow a hypothesis to be generated through the experience of practice itself. Once an observation is made or a hypothesis proposed, it can then be examined, tested, and modified through the practice of critical acceptance.

To be clear, set sequences are not intrinsically prescriptive, since they may be taught in a number of different ways, just as variable sequences may be taught from a rigidly prescribed perspective. What is encouraged herein is the ongoing evaluation of theory at the foundation of one's teaching, and the concomitant methods and techniques used to develop, elucidate, and practice this theory. It is the contention of this book that prescriptive methods inhibit learning, encouraging instead rote imitation and a lack of questioning. This, in turn, creates a disciplinary culture that is inflexible and stagnant.

In addition to the descriptive presentation of useful theoretical information (embodiment, kinesiology, ritual, aesthetics) the decision was made to depersonalise this presentation. A book about teaching by two long-time yoga practitioners/teachers has by necessity been informed by personal experience; however, with rare exception this book does not include the authors' personal stories, struggles, or revelations. Instead, it presents the results of ongoing experimentation as a critical enterprise, and challenges teachers and aspiring teachers to do the same. This book does not provide sample sequences, standard adjustments, mantras, class themes, or other templates of any kind. It does, however, provide resources meant to give individual teachers the agency to do so for themselves – through a novel presentation of perspectives from seemingly disparate disciplines, open-ended exercises meant to illustrate the concepts described, and an emphasis on critical inquiry and creative problem solving. It asks yoga teachers to be excellent through an active scepticism that looks for demonstrable truths that can be replicated through physical experimentation. In short, it follows other truth-seeking disciplines through the application of the scientific method for the advancement of disciplinary knowledge.

THE CONTENT OF THE BOOK

Chapter One: The Physical Philosophy of Yoga: Asana and Vinyasa

This chapter introduces the idea that the practice of yoga is an aesthetic creation, which is used as a technology that attempts to comprehend the ineffable. It explores how natural phenomena have been studied from the time of the pre-Socratics and Kapila and how this has developed into both the modern scientific method and contemporary aesthetics. The concepts of *purusha* and *prakriti* are described in a modern context through concepts used in artistic exploration. The differences between *asana* and *vinyasa* are distinguished and contemporary philosophies are articulated for each. Emphasis is placed on physical experimentation as a mechanism for discovery and testing philosophical hypotheses and is described as *physical philosophy*. Through these conjectures, yoga is defined as the study of the *Self* and its relation to "reality".

Chapter Two: Teaching Yoga: Methodology, Meaning, and Ritual

This chapter describes both tools and theoretical perspectives through which teachers may construct a robust methodology by framing the practice and teaching of yoga as a ritual progression. Through ritual, practitioners make meaning of their experiences as they struggle with material until it can be integrated logically into a larger belief system; one that explains their place in relation to the nature of reality (worldview). As the ritual operator, the successful teacher relies on their ability to structure lessons, so that students may find meaning in what are otherwise routine or ambiguous actions and experiences. The stages of ritual progression are described from the anthropological perspective and examined in the context of yoga classes and training.

Chapter Three: Teaching Somatic Practices of Yoga: Theory, Method, Technique, and Form

This chapter presents tools that provide the foundational knowledge required to teach any style of physical yoga and reviews the principal components of body dynamics. The relationship between mind and body is discussed in an overview of embodiment theory, fundamentals of kinesiology, and principles of movement. The concept of *levels* is considered through the theory of *pedagogical approximation* – the alignment of lessons to the knowledge base of students. A detailed discussion of the four basic components of teaching – *theory, method, technique,* and *form* – is introduced, described, and their hierarchical relationship established. The chapter concludes with applications of theoretical perspectives on teaching and learning.

Chapter Four: The Business of Yoga: To Teach or Not to Teach

This chapter looks at the impact that the popularity of yoga has had on the profession of teaching, the emergence of the "industry of yoga", and the proliferation of teacher training programmes. The various ways yoga has become aligned with social institutions (medicine, fitness, spirituality) are discussed along with the effects this has had on the way practitioners view the practice, the efficacy, and the uses of yoga. The ideal of "community" as a way of defining yoga both globally and locally is critically evaluated. The difficulties of sustaining a career in yoga teaching, both practically (concerning time, interest, and stamina) and financially, are addressed. The distinctions between teacher, practitioner, and student are articulated to clarify the different demands of each role.

Chapter Five: The Effective Yoga Teacher: Finding Your Voice

The chapter begins with a discussion of what is meant by persona, speech, and voice. *Voice* is refined through a process of discovery and then employed to express one's *persona*. The danger surrounding inauthentic voices of teachers and gurus is critically examined through controversies within the yoga community. The meta-message in one's *speech* is shown to be interpreted through the various aspects of the teacher's presentation, particularly through their use of language. Practical skills such as building and maintaining a clientele, studio etiquette, and professional demeanour are outlined as is the importance of self-practice and its role in the teacher's development of empathy for students and their experiences. This chapter details the ways teachers manage and maintain an authentic voice while being cognisant of its impact.

Chapter Six: Critical Social Issues for Yoga Teachers: Borders and Boundaries

This chapter discusses the dynamics of power within the yoga studio and other teaching contexts. The status and role of teacher and student are examined through behavioural strategies found in the manipulation of territory and personal space. The implications of dominance and submission and how they are employed appropriately in the teaching context are considered. The importance of creating and maintaining appropriate boundaries is noted as is the violation of these boundaries (the critical issue of "somatic dominance"). The authority exerted by organisations, teachers, studio cultures, and "tribal" membership is critically examined as is its impact on teaching. Particular consideration is given to the meaning of touch, the important role of touch, and the future of touch in the context of yoga teaching.

Chapter Seven: The Future of Practice

Yoga has been a discipline reliant on the teachings of the past; its evolution, however, will entail that it embraces new developments in the future. This chapter imagines the future of yoga in light of technological advancement, scientific discoveries, and cultural changes. The future of the "yoga studio" and the way teaching will be delivered is considered as are the pros and cons of classes, courses, workshops, and training formats. The prospects offered by new technologies for both teaching and the performance of yoga are explored, and aesthetic possibilities are imagined. The conditions for creating a legacy of the modern practice are reviewed. The chapter concludes with an appeal for continued critical inquiry and the recognition of the necessity of embodied, embedded "research" by teachers and practitioners who wish to investigate and to further the discipline's evolution.

Appendices: Reflection and Experimentation

The exercises presented at the end of each chapter provide ideas for reflection and experimentation. These shed light on the theoretical presentation of the text, provide practical techniques for cultivating critical acceptance, and encourage teachers to express their own, well researched, ideas. These exercises are open ended; they can be expanded, have no single answer or resolution, and can be returned to repeatedly. They are intended for both the practitioner and the teacher and provide ways to link knowledge gained through personal practice to the practice of teaching.

CRITICAL ISSUES

Although yoga may be practiced simply as a system of fitness or general well-being, it is the premise of this book that yoga can be more; a path for discovering larger truths. Framed this way, yoga is a serious discipline, and, as such, must deal directly with difficult issues that threaten to derail legitimacy. Contemporary yoga is a worldwide phenomenon, having spread from its origins in Eastern (if not "Indian") cultures.[1] As such, it has gone through a process of syncretism,[2] wherein its practices and interpretations have been modified to fit into the worldview of the receiving culture (as with all practices and beliefs that undergo the process of diffusion).[3] These changes are not viewed herein as "heretical" but rather as exemplary of an ongoing and eternal process; as Andrea Jain (2015) notes, yoga has always accommodated the context in which it is practiced. This process of testing and reimagining results in the strengthening and refining of ideas, rather than their corruption. It is the position of this book that varied cultural insights should be acknowledged for both their contributions and circumscribed perspectives; they are culturally specific ways of making sense of yoga as a practice in line with an existing set of beliefs.

In addition, what may seem like mundane issues, like the social dynamics of classroom interaction, building a clientele, and the meaning of corrections, are discussed along with more difficult, yet pressing, concerns such as the maintenance of boundaries, the acceptance of conspiracy theories, and what has come to be called *somatic dominance*. All are discussed in detail in an effort to highlight the importance of these issues, and the need for teachers to engage with difficult subjects. These subjects are so central to the vocation of teaching that a teacher avoids them at their own peril. Yet, they are rarely, if ever, broached in teacher training texts. This book provides a way to begin these discussions.

EMBEDDED AND EMBODIED

The production of knowledge in every culture is accomplished through experimentation. Though "science" is often imagined as an enterprise that produces quantitative data, this book, by contrast, avers the importance of qualitative data borne through experience;[4] the principle on which yogic knowledge is based. Any form of participant observation[5] requires that the researcher be both embodied and embedded in their experimental setting. Rather than being anecdotal (a misplaced, yet often cited critique), this method produces knowledge that has a high degree of validity – the research site and variables are not controlled (as they are in the laboratory setting) because all the data is significant.[6] Within this framework, a research topic evolves and is honed through the experience of experimentation. It reveals itself naturally out of the peaked interest of the participant researcher, whose body is an essential instrument for study. The greatest enemy to experimentation is the preconceptions of the researcher yogi, whose insights risk constraint by their bias. This is why, like an anthropologist, the yogi, interested in understanding the unknown, must acknowledge the discoveries of the past, but remain cognisant of their existing beliefs as they immerse themselves in somatic exploration. Critical acceptance and the physical philosophy that ensues from embedded, embodied research encourages such introspection, and honours the renegades throughout history who have suspended their beliefs in order to advance our understanding of the ephemeral.

Notes

1 The notion of "nation-states" is a modern concept created centuries after the origins of yoga and other exploratory techniques. Likewise, recent research questions whether even Hindu origin is accurate, since the oldest known postural texts are Buddhist in origin (Mallinson 2020).
2 Syncretism is the combination or merging of varying beliefs and practices. See Carl W. Ernst (April 2005). Here, Ernst discusses the way that the Sufis (an Islamic mystical tradition) have adapted yogic techniques to their own spiritual ends.
3 Diffusion is the movement of a trait from one culture or area to another. Diffusion always involves the syncretism of traditions in an effort to make the adopted practice fit into the worldview of the adopting culture.
4 Quantitative research produces numerical data (things that may be counted or quantified). Qualitative research, by contrast, produces descriptive data that is not easily reduced to quantification (ranking, precise measurement).
5 Originating in the field of anthropology, the ethnographic method of participant observation was created to ensure that cultural understanding emerged through direct embodied experience within a fieldsite. This experience involved the dual actions of participating in the everyday activities of the culture while simultaneously observing these same activities. Fieldwork differed from "armchair" research in that it required the observation of phenomenon in their natural environment.
6 *Validity* is a scientific term that measures how well research findings reflect the reality they claim to represent. Since the participant researcher is observing phenomenon as they naturally occur, their data of natural phenomena are more likely to show validity than in manipulated and constrained research settings.

References

Dewey, John. *How we think: a restatement of the relation of reflective thinking to the educative process.* Boston: D.C. Heath and company, 1933.
Ernst, Carl W. "Situating Sufism and yoga." *Journal of the Royal Asiatic Society* (April 2005): 15–43.

Jain, Andrea. *Selling yoga: from counterculture to pop culture.* New York: Oxford University Press, 2015.

Mallinson, James. *James Mallinson on Tantric traditions and Haṭhayoga.* Video, Brown University, 19 April, 2019. Accessed, 8 February, 2020. www.youtube.com/ watch?v=eUD2ni2U890.

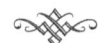

CHAPTER ONE

THE PHYSICAL PHILOSOPHY OF YOGA
ASANA AND VINYASA

AESTHETIC PHILOSOPHY

Aesthetic philosophy is a study of sensual perception, the way we evaluate beauty, and the significance this has for appreciating reality. " 'Aesthetics' deriving from the Greek word aesthesis ('perception'), was coined by the German philosopher, Alexander Baumgarten, in the middle of the eighteenth century. By it he meant 'the science of sensory knowledge', though the term soon began to be confined to a particular area of such knowledge and understood as 'the science of sensory beauty'" (Cooper 1997, 1). Grounded in processing sensory information, aesthetic appreciation is essential for the way physical yoga is used to decipher material reality, but also has a bearing on understanding the transcendent. The aesthetics of contemporary physical yoga practice are considered here by examining two major technical approaches – one that works through approximate stillness and one that attempts continuous fluid movement. The prospects and propositions of yoga, based on stillness, form a large part of the textual canon, though the actual techniques for accomplishing it lack definitive clarity. There is also considerable writing on the nature of "action", which has some bearing on the way that movement can be done yogically. In modern practice, stillness is generally associated with

DOI: 10.4324/9781003181910-2

asana and movement with *vinyasa* and these terms will be used loosely throughout to denote which of these approaches is being discussed.

The historical philosophies of yoga are indisputably important, however, when viewed without circumspection, they can become an impediment to the living evolution of yoga's practices and philosophy. The aphoristic style of ancient texts encourages interpretation, but these interpretations, when put into practice, appear rooted in the assumption that the profound questions yoga raises have already been adequately answered. The explorations of physical yoga are a vital and living quest for additional perspective; informed by new and provoking information and which are continuously subject to revision. The philosophical presentation of this chapter conveys the authors' experiences and comprehension of the practice and teaching of yoga (since the 1970s). It proposes a theory (later chapters suggest methods and techniques to investigate it) to explain these experiences and examines these through a variety of aesthetic and historical reflections on the nature of reality. The debates surrounding the ineffable, ancient, and complex philosophic traditions ascribed to yoga are rich in conjecture and remain unresolved. The aesthetic philosophy presented below is a way of making sense of this fascinating debate from a modern, Western, scientific perspective rather than an abandonment of the precepts of yogis from previous generations.

YOGA AND RELIGION

Philosophy taught from a physical perspective might be considered problematic. In the contemporary yoga studio setting, philosophy has been conflated with aspects of religion or else as something that has more to do with discussion than demonstration. It is worthwhile to begin by considering how religion and philosophy differ.

Religions have some orientation to unseen realms, beings, and powers; religion posits the existence of supernatural things (Stark and Bainbridge 1985, 3). Belief in these supernatural entities need not be proved or might belie demonstration. One of the demands of philosophy, in contrast, is that tenets must be logically derived and that the mechanism by which it obtains conclusions is demonstrable. David Lewis-Williams and David Pearce construct a useful paradigm to explain religion that, in many ways, fits well with an explanation of yoga. There are three mutually supporting aspects to be considered: *experience, belief,* and *practice*. They argue that "*Religious experience* is a set of mental states created by the functioning of the human brain in natural and induced conditions" and that people interpret these experiences as some "sort of contact with supernatural, but to them very real, realms … *Religious belief* derives, in the first instance, from attempts to codify this experience in specific social circumstances" (Lewis-Williams and Pearce 2005, 25–27).[1] Beliefs give meaning to religious experience. Religious practice refers to the way beliefs are manifested – the particular rituals and symbology of the society in which they occur. These practices are meant to lead people into religious experience and are a way of manifesting their beliefs. For instance, people may practice the belief that there is a heaven and hell by going to church on Sunday or that one can acquire spiritual insight by attending a yoga class once a week. The mystical experience is strengthened and affirmed because others attending share these convictions and is reinforced through symbology and practices (an *Om* sign on the door of the studio; a cross on the church – kneeling to pray or bringing the hands into *namaste*). The most profound mystical experiences in religion and yoga are rare, yet they are accorded validity through these beliefs and practices.

Philosophy asks difficult questions to which it posits hypothetical possibilities, whereas religion provides absolute answers, often supported by a canon of written or oral texts. Philosophy proposes and tests hypotheses, seeking to refine, refute, or reify the understanding of its subject. In physical yoga, philosophical hypotheses are tested through experience and conclusions are subject to revision. As the circumstances of a yoga posture change from day to day, the uniqueness of each experience is highlighted. Through ongoing experimentation, the practitioner tries to extrapolate – both about the particularity of the physical experience and what the meaning of this might be.

There is nothing in yoga practice that demands belief in supernatural beings, nor is there a necessity that the supernatural exist, although it has certainly been placed in a religious context in past analyses (Eliade 1958, 363).[2] While yoga may share some features of religion and make reference to celestial or supernatural beings, these are culturally specific (theistic) interpretations and are nonessential for the study of yoga and its physical philosophy (Jakubczak 2014). This is not to say that faiths are trivial for the individuals that hold them – on the contrary, religious beliefs may be useful for contextualising what an individual uniquely experiences through yoga.

EARLY NON-THEISTIC EXPLANATIONS OF THE FOUNDATIONS OF REALITY

Alternative and nontheistic views of yoga philosophy were derived during what Karl Jaspers refers to as the Axial Age (Jaspers 1955, 1–6). During the period of approximately eighth–second century BCE, a new way of conceiving reality flowered, as is found in the pre-Socratic philosophers of Greece and Kapila and the Buddha in the Indian subcontinent. This period marked the development of the notion that the cosmos was something that could be intellectually considered, and its unfolding pierced in ways that would show its workings through provable means. Natural phenomena would have demonstrable causes. Religious doctrine was no longer considered the sole means of construing reality. Milesian pre-Socratics, for example, sought to describe a reality that was conceived as a primal, indivisible unity from which natural phenomena appeared. Thales and Anaximenes, respectively, postulated that water and air were the elemental substances from which everything was derived. Anaximander imagined this unity as something he termed the *apeiron* – an entity without boundary; limitless – an early articulation of infinity of both space and time. Heraclitus (from Ephesus and at odds with the Milesians) maintained that it was not a substance, but rather, an ever-changing process, and his expression of this idea is that *one cannot step into the same river twice, for different waters flow by.*[3] These pre-Socratics contributed to the study of natural, rather than supernatural, phenomena as a means to understanding the nature of reality – something that matured through later Greek philosophy and which continues to evolve.

Richard Tarnas, in *The Passion of The Western Mind*, summarises the Greek philosophy that the pre-Socratics engendered as resulting in two philosophic strands – Platonic and Aristotelian (Tarnas 1991, 69–71). The Platonic seeks hidden/mystical truths through the use of reason and presupposes an ordered cosmos, which analysis reveals as a timeless order that is both rational and mythic. The Aristotelian relies on what the five senses can discern and demands that theoretical understanding be measured against empirical reality. The mythological and supernatural – undemonstrable otherworld realities – are excluded from causal explanations. One of the dynamic tensions here is the theoretical assumption of "mystical truths" in the Platonic tendency and the Aristotelian exclusion of "undemonstrable otherworld realities". The following examples illustrate the contention that yoga is an aesthetic philosophy that seeks to understand reality through physical means. Consider the beauty of the stars or planets shining in the sky – Venus for example. There it is – named for a deity – visibly glowing brighter than the rest in the twilight or early morning. The Platonic view might be something like: "Ah yes, an example of beauty, but not something that fully epitomises the complete ideal of beauty. However, we can calculate through mathematical formulae the exact trajectory of its course through the sky and come to the conclusion that these formulae reveal a profound structure of elegant and knowable harmony to be found in this natural phenomenon that can be extrapolated to larger or smaller structures – that the nature of the universe and of beauty is to be found in this exactitude." The Aristotelian view would be that: "It is glowing the way it does in the twilit sky because the atmosphere is 'just so' on this occasion and it is being viewed from a particular vantage point – its beauty lies in a combination of many factors that create the unique way it appears on this occasion." If we change the example from Venus to a yoga student executing a posture or sequence, a teacher, of a Platonic perspective, might be viewing it to see how well it conforms to their ideal of the form (its "sacred geometry") or an Aristotelian might be looking to find what factors are making it occur as it does on this particular occasion (the warmth of the room and student's physical anatomy). In both cases, the summary of the details is meant to return the analysis to something larger. One perspective holds that there are precise alignments of body parts etc. that point to an understanding and congruence with a Platonic "mystical plane – a music of the spheres". The other believes that this is an Aristotelian phenomenon – a unique occurrence, and that in the sum of the details of the experience exists an explanation of reality.

While the pre-Socratic philosophers pondered primal substance and process, the Vedic sage Kapila proposed two categories of reality – *prakriti* and *purusha*.[4] Prakriti is, basically, "matter"; the stuff/substance that comes into "being". As "matter", the nature of *prakriti* is impermanent – ever-changing, forever dissolving and reassembling itself – an endless atomistic alteration. In contrast, *purusha* is characterised as unchanging, but *purusha* is less susceptible to easy definition – though, vernacularly, it has been described as "spirit" or "consciousness". Exactly what Kapila, in his cultural milieu, might have construed it to be is speculative, but modern interpretations of *purusha* involve the idea that a person's spirit is totally distinct from their material self and endeavour to account for both its immateriality and its reality. The analysis that follows uses the word "potential" to describe this. It is real because it could happen (not impossible), but immaterial because it has not become manifest. This is in accord with the pre-Socratics' interest in cause and effect. Like the proto science of the pre-Socratics, this provides a way to look at cause and effect; the actions performed in *prakriti*[5] bring the potential inherent in *purusha* into material being. If water, for example, was heated it would turn to steam; the action of heat brought it into being, but water could not become blood by heating it because that is not something that is latent in *purusha*; as a potentiality it does not exist – it is not real.

Objections could be made against "potentiality" as a description of *purusha*. Traditionally, *purusha* has been described as "pure consciousness" (the "spirit" or "person" that is a passive attribute of living creatures), a mere inactive spectator, a state of indifference, irreducible, without qualities, free from engagement with *prakriti*. It is something that *buddhi* (intelligence) cannot know because, even as a highly evolved part of *prakriti*, it can only know other parts of *prakriti*. Furthermore, the only way to know this "pure consciousness" is to wholly overcome life – dying to be reborn, if taken literally. It is impossible to corroborate the state of *purusha* empirically through *prakriti*. Also, traditionalists might wonder how "potentiality" accounts for an irreducible "I" – a kind of inactive observer who is eternal and unchanged, everlasting consciousness. It may be impossible to adequately describe with words (products of *buddhi*) and exactitude this "reality". Nevertheless, the concept "potentiality" does provide a starting point for modern practitioners' investigations into understanding the nature of "pure consciousness" through yoga.

Potentiality does satisfy a number of the conditions ascribed to *purusha*. Potentiality is indifferent to whether it becomes realised. It is simply a fact – it could happen, but it has no interest in making it happen. As an infinite vastness of amorphous contingency, it is unattached – it cannot facilitate or influence its own coming into being. That is the role of "cause"; something in *prakriti*. Having no substance, it is irreducible. The essential "I" of each "person" or "spirit", being irreducible, shares this reality with all "persons" or "spirits" so that, even though a person may die, this essentiality carries on. Pure consciousness would be everlasting in this sense. Though Samkhya philosophy applies this to living creatures, it is not a stretch to think that this same potentiality could be extended to the inanimate. *Purusha* is something that is real, but not material, nor is it spatially or temporally bound. "Potential" does fit these requirements.

MATERIAL REALITY AS ILLUSION

What relevance does this have for the yogi and physical philosophy? One might propose that people engage in actions, and through their actions they take what is latent and make it manifest in *prakriti*. In yoga philosophy, "action" is understood as *karma* and has a number of nuanced interpretations. It means "cause and effect", "physical movement" (Nyaya-Upanishads), the "transitory rather than permanent feature of that which it creates, or any activity performed in the course of material existence" (Bhaktivedanta Narayana Gosvami Maharaja and Bhaktivinoda Ṭhākura 2015). In his early analysis of yogis in India, Mircea Eliade described things that were manifest through cause and effect as *maya* –fleeting impressions accorded validity, but which were illusory. Practitioners believed that a single, everlasting, and unchanging unity was the true nature of existence and that ignorance of an unchanging, foundational Self could be overcome through the practice of yoga.[6]

Though much is speculative when considering the contemplative and active pursuits of ancient minds and cultures, one foundational premise of early yogic principles is that the individual can come to experience this condition of a reality that appears to be *other* than that which appears *evident*. The "illusion" of separateness was seen as the individual's mistaken belief that their own life was the true reality. To overcome this *maya*, yogis practised extreme austerities to master the body and the mind's dependence on sensual input – endeavouring to look "inwards" to find that which was foundational in the universe. In other words, they sought a negation of "self", which they saw either as an impediment to understanding or the cause of the illusion of separateness from the great unity[7]. To achieve mastery – to effect substantial and lasting change – they put themselves into intense situations (standing on one leg or holding the arm in the air until the muscles wither; remaining motionless under the blazing hot sun). Postures would be held for hours or, at its most extreme, for years. This pursuit of extreme postures and exposure to extreme situations was presumably done in the belief that overcoming the embodied self in fairly benign circumstances did not guarantee success under duress and that the effects were less palpable.

This required an unflinching commitment to the exploration of ceasing to identify with the body and personality – an effort to bring about an experience of "no action", changelessness.

A PHILOSOPHY FOR *VINYASA*

One of the fascinating developments in modern yoga has been the rise of *vinyasa* (Birch 2018, 101–180).[8] Despite its popularity, no extensive philosophy for its techniques and workings has yet been articulated. Modern and traditional yoga have emphasised the techniques of asana – the "stable seat" of postural yoga – valourising it as essential for contemplative pursuits. *Vinyasa*, instead, considers the transitions between postures to be of equal import – at its most extreme, eliminating posture altogether and advocating continuous fluid movement, which is motivated by, and synchronised with, breath. Historically, *asana* yoga techniques attempt to simulate a deep experience of changelessness. The body is held immobile, suspended breathing (a refinement on bodily immobility) is valued and effort is made to arrest the workings of the mind by bringing it to a point of fixity – essentially negating mundane bodily process to achieve a more lucid experience of the unity that it sees as the true nature of the universe. Eliade says, "... determined and continuous concentration, called *ekagrata* ('on a single point'), is obtained by integrating the mental flux ... which dams the mental stream and thus constitutes a 'psychic mass', a solid and unified continuum" (Eliade 1958, 47–48). This possibly shares the concerns of the Milesian pre-Socratic philosophers in their efforts to determine the true nature of the universe as a foundational or primordial substance.

Vinyasa, in this analysis, however, shares a more Heraclitian notion – it posits that the foundation is a process rather than a substance. It chooses the evenness with which the process unfolds as its *ekagrata* rather than the fixity on a single and immovable point. *Vinyasa's* techniques involve sustaining evenness of breath and synchronising this with evenness of the body's movement to create evenness of mind; though it could be argued that evenness of mind is actually the first requirement. Most likely, the breath, body, and mind are involved in a dynamically reciprocal arrangement.

The *vinyasa* techniques assume that time flows at an even rate so that there are no "moments" of greater import. There are other possible theories for the flow of time: it could be evenly accelerating; slowing; or flowing erratically. A fourth possibility is that there is no such thing as time – it is merely an abstract convention for an eternal and undifferentiated present that is simultaneously brought into being and annihilated – something that, paradoxically, is unity through its unceasing changingness. To develop awareness of this unceasing flow, effort is made to sustain a lengthened breath. Postures are moved through and accorded no more importance than the movement coming towards them or away again. Because there is a differentiation when the breath changes from inhale to exhale and back again, there is a sense that duration *does* have some importance, and this would incline one away from the notion above that there is no such thing as time. The length of a breath does provide a very practical limit for the development of focus or concentration – it is a comparatively short time to hold one's focus. When it is over, there is little attachment to one's experience for there is little investment in it and the next breath, with its own challenges, follows swiftly. Each breath is unique and savoured for what it is and what is revealed in its duration. The process begins anew with each breath and there is no fidelity to the breath past or the breath to come.

When it is said that breathing is synchronised with movement, it means more than "they happen at the same time". Each breath is meant to be full; yet controlled without undue strain. The movement accompanying it is likewise – that particular breath could only produce the movement that it does – the movement tries to be a perfect rendition of what that breath is – not just as it happens in time, but also sharing its qualities. And, likewise with the mind – it is in perfect accord with the breath. If the breath is slightly ragged, it would indicate a like agitation in the mind. The breath is considered an accurate intermediary between physical and mental processes; each part mediating and endeavouring to accurately reflect the state of the whole as it moves through an ongoing transitional process. This *vinyasa* philosophy proposes an alternative to *asana*'s search for the perfection of stillness, arguing that regardless of how intently an *asana* practitioner attempts to remain still, their breathing must inevitably result in a measure of movement. Furthermore, while the body appears relatively still in *asana*, blood continues to course through it, cells continue to replicate and die, and the endocrine system continues to function. From the right vantage point, the *asana* yogi would be seen as sitting on a planet that spins on its axis as it hurtles around the sun – a sun that is situated in an evolving and slowly rotating galaxy, which is in an expanding universe (Rees 2001, 50–51).[9] In short, the nature of reality is this process of movement and change, and that, to be one with it, it is necessary to attune oneself to this process.

There are other notable differences between *asana* and *vinyasa*. The practitioners of *asana*, in ultimately seeking detachment from bodily sensation – exposing themselves to extreme physical trials until mastery is achieved in stillness – "look" inwardly in the search for the unity of foundational Self. The *vinyasa* technique posited here, however, uses a style of *ujjayi* breathing to begin energetically at an infinitely small point within the pelvic area from which it moves outwardly with a unity of breath, body, and mind. Before discussing the significance of inward and outward, the terms *prana* and *pranayama* (the yogic terms for energy and techniques used for its movement) should be clarified. The meaning of *prana,* and therefore *pranayama,* is ambiguous. Eliade describes prana as "organic energy discharged by inhalation and exhalation" (Eliade 1958, 58) without defining what that organic energy is or where it goes. A popular contemporary definition is *vital life force energy,* though it is unclear whether the adjective vital means there are other forms of life force energy. Swami Rama suggests that *prana* permeates all reality including inanimate objects (Rama 2002, 202). This broad definition might indicate that *prana* could be energy such as that found at an atomic level. The term *yama* is sometimes defined as "restraint", but "control" or "manipulation" are also terms that could be applied.[10] In *asana* yoga, there is an endeavour to bring the *prana* into a state where there is no flux – no discharge of energy. The *Hatha Yoga Pradipika* (Sinh 1915, 4.18) and the *Siva Samhita* (Vasu 1914–15, 2.13) enumerate the channels called *nadis* (72,000 and 350,000 respectively) in the body through which *prana* travels. James Mallinson and Mark Singleton in their *Roots Of Yoga* review the idea that the main *nadis* begin at the "base" *chakra* and move to the "crown" *chakra* (top of the head), enabling *prana* to move through the "subtle body" (Mallinson and Singleton 2017, 171–184). The idea of a mysterious source of energy commencing near the base of the spine with attached channels through which energy rises is a premise, so pervasive and staunchly held, that one has to step well back to get perspective on what an extraordinary and peculiar assertion this is if taken literally – predicated on "subtle bodies" with elaborate structures that belie demonstration, and yet, which have apparently resonated with practitioners through the ages; replete with ethical, epistemological, and aesthetic concerns. The "lower" *chakras* (nexuses of *pranic* energy) are baser and more instinctual; the higher ones have more noble and spiritual import; lower ones are more simplistic in their features and the higher more detailed in their elaboration. The degree to which these purported structures should be taken literally in practice is open to debate. They are, however, powerful tools for the imagination and have both poetic and metaphoric resonance.

The *vinyasa* philosophy presented here argues that the "subtle body" and its structures do not stand up to literal interpretation. *Vinyasa*, however, loosely follows this energetic premise and conceives of it as imagery that works well as a metaphoric device for its *ekagrata* of continuous flow. This imagery is uniquely conceived and practised by each individual and is a useful poetic conception around which the *vinyasi* can cohesively integrate the concrete efforts of body, mind, and breath. Whatever form one might conceive of a *nadi,* and an energy that travels through it, it is likely that each individual imagines it in their own way ("My *sushumna* is like a silvery thread"; "Mine is like a plastic tube"). The place where this energy begins is conceived of as the *mula* (though not as a *chakra*) and locates it as an infinitely small and imaginary, but conceptually potent, point located in the pelvic area situated somewhere between the sitting bones, the pubic bone, the coccyx, and the pelvic floor. This is the imagined point of origin of the outward flow of *prana*. Though an accepted translation of *mula* has been "root", this definition may miss some of the subtlety that "place or point of origin" would suggest.[11] The *vinyasa* imagery functions as a cogent focal point – its ekagrata – from which the body moves in a unified way. This conceit provides the structure to imagine moving *prana* (the action of *pranayama*) from this infinitely small point – so small that it amounts to the same as a zero point on a number line. *Mula* is the starting place of the sustained movement of energy both in the direction of the legs and feet and in the direction of the torso, the head, and the arms – likened to a light radiating outwards. Zero points on number lines and light radiating from infinitely small points should be recognised for what they are: culturally specific metaphors that attempt to provide analogies for an experience that will be uniquely construed by each practitioner. The facility for imaginative engagement with the experience is important to this theory of *vinyasa* – just as important as intellectual, emotional, and physical engagement. The entirety of one's being is dedicated to the experience.

On the face of it, both *asana* and *vinyasa* seem to hold extreme polar positions – one a complete negation of self and the other a full affirmation, but both are predicated on the entry (or rebirth) into a different sphere of being or experience – that of understanding the true nature of reality. A mastery of technique is the means by which they try to ensure their ability to recapture the experience at will. In this effort, each has difficult obstacles to surmount. In *asana* – for those looking inwardly – the multiple distractions of their own thoughts must be quelled as they aspire to find a different and more universal plane of experience. For those looking outwardly, there is the difficulty of incorporating all that their senses bring them and responding to this in a wholly cogent way – one that sees the blatant manifestation of a unique and evolving "other" with which they are trying to meld their understanding. *Vinyasa* recognises that each individual does this as an imaginative and uniquely creative enterprise, and this places it in the purview of aesthetic philosophy.

Sensory Control

In this theory of *vinyasa*, *pratayahara* refers to the relationship of the senses to the mind. Though it does figure in some way in most classes of modern yoga, it is not something that is often referred to by name. For *vinyasa*, there are three working definitions of its processes. The first and most standard one is "sense withdrawal". Techniques might involve working with the eyes shut and the point of this is to eliminate the possible distractions of the visual sense. Yoga done on a mat also works in this way – by confining the space in which the practice takes place, it lessens the impact of sensual information that comes from beyond it. A second definition might be "sense refinement". For example, *vinyasa's* effort to sustain movement can be aided by sensual information. As one moves one's arm and hands through space, the subtle feeling of air passing between the fingers can be detected. Though subtle, the sensation between the fingers gives a clear metering of exactly how smooth the movement is. It should be noted that there is some crossover between these two definitions. If you close your eyes to do a practice, other sensual information becomes more prominent. The third definition of *pratayahara* is "rethinking" or "thinking otherwise". Phulgenda Sinha suggests that "when the mind is disturbed by improper thoughts the remedy is to contemplate the opposite".[12] For example, the distractions created by concentrating on the many body parts needed to perform *vinyasa* can be overcome by instead imagining oneself as an energetic singularity radiating outwards.

Focused Concentration

The term *dharana* denotes the act of concentration on a "single point" or *ekagrata*. The volume of this single point is important – it could be conceived as a dot (or infinitely larger or smaller) as well as an internal space (such as between the brows – the third eye). The practitioner makes effort to dedicate the whole of their being to fill or encompass this singularity. As the size and shape of the ekagrata is variable, external objects for contemplation can as easily be a lotus blossom as a dot on paper. Internally, the size with which anyone conceives the third eye (or where exactly it is placed) is individual. The idea of volume is an important one in *vinyasa*. The *vinyasa* practitioner, in their involvement with external stimuli, seeks to expand the volume of consciousness to the limit of their capabilities in the circumstances of the place where they practise and refers to this process as *dhyana*.

In the performing arts, *dhyana* is something that is regularly practised. For actors, their work must be appropriately scaled to fit the theatre. They "project" their performance to fit the space. The volume of their consciousness is the size of the theatre. If they are distracted by someone coughing in the third row, that becomes the size of the space of their awareness (and the performance suffers). This whole process begins early in rehearsal as they first craft a reality between their fellow actors, which gradually expands to adequately fill the rehearsal room. Most laypeople believe that an actor assumes an emotional attitude; that they play, for instance, the emotion of sadness. But this is not how it is done. Instead, the audience gets the impression of a character *being* sad because, over the course of a number of simple and specific "actions", the actor develops the audience's intuition – "I pick up the teacup ... bring it to my lips ... put it down untasted" – and the accumulation of these individual actions makes the impression. In theatre, these individual moments are selected and executed in a way that is, for the most part, unlike real life. They are done with a single focus. This singularity of focus is very much the kind of single pointed concentration that is practised in *vinyasa* yoga as it transitions through postures.

Like the actor with the teacup, the *vinyasi* attempts to structure their practice with a series of approximately reproducible actions. During each inhalation and each exhalation, only one action is accomplished. An inhalation might be the move to a high arch, an exhalation the move from a high arch to a forward bend. If one looks at any individual part of the body, essentially there is only one movement. In the case of the high arch, the arms might describe a single arc; the pelvis would only move forward; the rib cage expand uniformly – and these movements happen at exactly the rate of the breath so that their maximal movement is reached at the same time. Each breath, and the movement it engenders, is also a clear record of the mind. Someone who is over-eager to emulate a high arch they have admired, may rush to get the arms further back than the breath would predicate. The ephemeral and fleeting nature of mind (or spirit) and the body (matter) are both aspects of the same reality and each breath provides a window on an individual's engagement with that reality.

The practise of *dhyana* illustrates how space or volume reciprocally work to affect the practitioner. Things that are not "of" the individual – that which is "other" – influence the way the practitioner experiences reality. A cold room has an effect on the way movement is evoked. The individual also changes the space. The effort of their movement, for instance, slightly heats the room – their "energy" alters "the other". In the case of an actor playing a sad scene, the energy committed to the conception of the volume of their consciousness (a theatre space) will cause someone sitting in the back row to also feel sad (regardless of whether the circumstances of their life are happy or otherwise).

In a yoga studio, the volume of consciousness may be constrained or expanded in various ways. The use of rectangular yoga mats is nearly ubiquitous and is a modern addition to yoga practice. While they provide cushioning and traction, they also, for many, limit their relationship to space – providing a barrier that insulates from intrusion, but that also inhibits expansion beyond. Many students will scramble about to ensure that their feet, or hands, or head never come off the mat. There are factors that may mitigate this. For instance, if a studio is spacious, it creates a tendency to draw one's awareness into the space; and the use of music has the potential to draw forth a more expansive relationship between the practitioner and whatever "space" the music suggests.

The Between Space

There appears to be a field (*Between Space*) in which the operations of the "actor's sadness" or the yoga practitioner's experience with "the other" occur. What is the *Between Space*? Theoretically, the volume of consciousness could be infinite; boundless like the *apeiron* of the pre-Socratics. It is a long way from the rectangle of a yoga mat to the edge of the perceivable universe. Even the relatively small distances of our immediate cosmic neighbourhood strain the imagination,[13] though that is one human tool for broaching such space. Science has managed this problem by quantifying it. Fourteen billion light years[14] does not seem that intimidating when viewed as words on a page. *Asana* practice would seem to posit that this vastness is the same as the volume to be found internally through the negation of thought-movements until there is an irreducible essence of negligible volume (that is also immaterial and temporally unbound) and that this foundation – the "essential self" – is the same as the universe. The idea that the infinitely small and the infinitely large are the same may seem counterintuitive, but there are possible rationales for this. For example, according to Big Bang Theory, the entirety of the vast universe emerged from a high density/high temperature single point. The *vinyasa* yogi's focus on the expansion of the volume of consciousness may be seen as a personal attempt to replicate this process whereas the *asana* yogi's looking inwards attempts to reverse time and space wherein the whole of the universe is withdrawn again into a single essential point that contains the All. Comparisons between physics and yoga are inevitably strained. The ambition of physical yoga practice may be equal to physics conjecturally but may be too constrained by the limitations of its "laboratory". Yet there remains the possibility that a prodigy *sadhu* could have had insights as seemingly improbable as Maxwell or Einstein's recognition that Newtonian physics, though having the appearance of common sense (space and time as absolutes), is not the actuality (that space and time are warped).

Definitive conclusions on how the modern scientific understanding of space affects the contemporary yogi's apprehension of "true reality" cannot yet be made – it can be tentatively accepted as a leap of faith that the world is not as we mundanely apprehend it. It is worthwhile to examine, with imperfect knowledge, what can be observed and gleaned from "life as it is lived". There are "*dhyanic*" aspects to the way a theatre audience's attention works in the *Between Space*. Their volume of consciousness must encompass what the actor is doing. A clearer illustration of the way volume of consciousness and the *Between Space* operate is found in the way a sunset is experienced. The grandeur of a sky extravagantly hued with coloured light and shadows playing on the clouds might inspire one to experience beauty. However, the experience of beauty does not exist if there is no one to see it (just as the sadness of the audience does not exist if there is no audience – the beauty and sadness are experiences; not things in and of themselves). The experience only happens when the participant has their volume of consciousness expanded to take in the scope – the *Between Space* – in which the experience is made to occur. There is no analysis of the experience – the participant is not considering whether those cumulonimbus clouds would be better if they were cirrus. There is acceptance and participation. As small as the role of the audience may seem, they have a part to play, for without them, the experience of beauty would not occur. The *vinyasi* plays the same role in the much larger sphere of the universe itself. The direct experience of the Totality may be what is meant by the term *samadhi*. For the union of yoga to be complete, there would have to be a dissolving of the sense that the person perceiving is distinct from the sunset – so that they exist without differentiation.[15] To believe this can be accomplished with the tool of imagination is a leap of faith.[16]

MIND AND AESTHETIC PHILOSOPHY

In his essays in *The Dance of Siva*, the philosopher Ananda K. Coomaraswamy makes the claim that the experiencing of beauty is the same as religious experience and that "we are justified in identifying beauty with Brahman – and that in this experience, the distinction between individual and Brahman is transcended." To articulate this, he presents a useful template for the "history" of any work of art; identifying the artistic process as (Coomaraswamy 1985, 30–45):

1. An intuition of matter/subject
2. Internal vision
3. Externalizing the vision into a technical vehicle
4. The stimulation of the perceiver.

The first three of these are the province of the artist and the fourth is the realm of the audience wherein the connection is made between the artist's vision and the perceiver who is given an insight into the nature of Beauty/Reality/*Brahman*. This is the moment when the aesthetic emotion is awakened in the viewer and has nothing to do with their analytic capacity. This emotion is the self-same experience of looking at a fabulous sunset. The observer is struck with a sudden awe at the magnitude of what they notice. There is a self-forgetting – a sharing of a unified existence.

If beauty can be discovered in anything because it latently exists in all things, an artist may find inspiration in any subject. Beethoven wrote about Elysian Fields – the Sex Pistols were interested in anarchy; Turner chose sky and Mondrian skyscrapers. They then rendered the subject in their own unique way as music or a painting. But beauty is neither in this technical rendering nor in its analytic associations for the observer. What is attractive to one observer is unattractive to another. Some like Beethoven and despise the Sex Pistols and vice-versa. Rather, beauty is in the moment of recognition – the awakening of aesthetic emotion in the perceiver. Beauty is the latent phase of *Brahman* that comes into being when this happens. The *vinyasa* aesthetic philosophy suggests this beauty is there to be perceived in all of reality.

As an aesthetic philosophy, *vinyasa's* position on using its technique to induce the experience of beauty is clear. The practitioner must have the technical capability to achieve their intention. A sunset, or a mountain, or a sculpture does not have to consider how to be the best sunset/mountain/sculpture it can be. It is what it is. The appreciation – or experience – of it comes from the creative input of the viewer. For the yoga practitioner, there is an odd situation where they are both viewer and the work of art – a living sculpture and appreciator. One implication is that each person will do their yoga in a way that is unique. Just as there is no ideal of a sunset to which all sunsets aspire, there is no version of a posture or rendering of a sequence that is ideal. The beauty would be experienced in the unique execution – a rendering that approximates something that is most essential in the person executing it – on a breath-by-breath basis. A posture performed as imitation is tainted or false – the "living sculpture" is trying to be something it is not. Someone straining for a backbend they are not anatomically capable of doing, or a hamstring stretch they do not have, is jarring to look at (and to feel) not just because it looks injurious, but also because there is a lack of congruence between the intention and the technical ability to render it. However much the lack of technical skill might be mitigated by appreciating enthusiastic effort, this is not the same as experiencing the wondrous awe of aesthetic emotion. The enthusiastic effort is predicated on *what could be* rather than *what is*. Appreciation functions to make clear *purusha's* existence by bringing it into being – making what was only potential, tangible. When viewing a skyscraper marvellously situated in its cityscape, one need not know what commerce goes on there or how it was constructed to experience beauty. So it is for the yoga practitioner whose technique is at one with their intention. Observing themselves, they do not need to know what a posture means, what health issue it might address, or whether it confers supernatural powers. It is beautiful because there is a congruency of intention, technical means, and rendering.

The aesthetic experience is not a measuring and weighing of details, but, rather, an intimation of the whole in which one is included. Such experiences give a unique perspective on the unity that the yogi seeks, but it is familiarity and an evaluation of detail that helps facilitate this. A beginner student might be intimidated when a more practised student demonstrates wrapping both legs behind the head or they might think that it just looks like something that hurts. As the beginner gains knowledge of yoga technique, they cease to simply consider the unusual flexibility the posture requires and instead begin to appreciate the relaxed demeanour of the body or the way the breath is being used in difficult circumstances and so evaluate it differently. Their aesthetic taste has changed because they have developed appreciation for more subtle aspects of yoga technique that reveal more of an intimation of the whole – the underlying nature of reality.

The Mind and Aesthetic Experience

What is this *prana* – this energy – that is both discharged and exchanged in the *Between Space* and what is its role in the experience of beauty? We might intuit that the heat released by the body, which slightly warmed the room, was the energy of that person. If that were so, at what point does it cease to be their energy – the moment it passes beyond the layer of the skin? Or, at what point did the energy first become a part of the yogi? When breathing, air is drawn into the lungs where it mingles with gas and tissue, from which oxygen is extracted and moved into the vascular system, where it is distributed throughout the body. At what point, if ever, did those oxygen molecules become part of the yogi? It should be obvious from these slightly facetious questions that there are three possibilities to entertain.

1. It is never part of the yogi.
2. It is transitorily part of the yogi.

3. There is no distinction between the yogi and energy – it is all one thing.

The hypothesis one chooses might confront the question of "What is the role of the mind in energy or *prana* manipulation?" As the "sad actor" example above suggests, through the process of mind, energy can be moulded and directed (and is palpably shown in the audience's reaction). The mind needs neurological function to exist, but it is not the same as a description of synapses and neurons or areas of the brain that can be mapped during stimulus just as it is not oxygen molecules. These are things through which mind operates. Mind is the process – a creative and malleable activity – and an influenceable one – which has proved difficult to quantify. Through the process of mind, the *vinyasa* yogi constructs a volume of consciousness through which they can influence the circumstances of that volume in the way the actor can make the audience members sad; without being able to say exactly how that sadness will be felt. The challenge for the *vinyasi* becomes one of how large they wish to make this sphere of influence. Through the process of mind, they create experience – they endeavour to reveal beauty through the exactitude with which they co-ordinate technique and intention. This is an aesthetic philosophy that is predicated on the idea that there is latent beauty to be experienced in the unfolding of the universe and that their role in it is creative as both doer and watcher.

Through enculturation, people develop aesthetic taste; they find or enhance appreciation for everything from food to lifestyle to art. Most experienced yoga practitioners have an "expert's" response the moment they see a yoga photograph or see yoga done in a studio because they recognise what the posture signifies in that moment; the range of yogic lifestyle and philosophy including its conceptions of the movement of energy. The posture is a concise reminder of some underlying truth and the moment of recognition – before analysis of meaning begins – is where the knowledge of beauty exists. The closer the rendering of the posture is to the "truth" of the posture, the more the observer is inclined to view it with satisfaction and not fret about its alignment or other aspects of technical execution. When something does not strike one as beautiful, it is often because the technical rendering of it is not sufficiently congruent with the content or intention. Art that stimulates the aesthetic emotion has a unity between technique and intention. Art and yoga are technologies that serve to create an aesthetic experience.

Yoga and Action

A supposition of art is that what it portrays gives insight – it frames a "vision" – it shows a perspective on reality; tries to somehow show the impossible. Likewise, the suppositions regarding the practice of yoga postures are that they reveal something ineffable. The practitioner tries to become wholly immersed in their actions – to go beyond working on a technique or considering what will happen next or reflecting on what has come before – to become both the work of art and the viewer. There is a congruency in their actions that moves the yogi to recognise the experience of the aesthetic emotion and to gain insight into the nature of the Totality; of *Brahman*.

The *Bhagavad Gita* has a particularly theatrical explanation of "action". Before a great battle, Arjuna is faced with an ethical dilemma. Though he is a warrior, and it is a "just" battle he is to fight, his despair at the immorality of killing his family members and mentors is unbearable. The solution to this problem is provided by his charioteer, Krishna (he is also a deity), who asserts that we become what our actions make us. As a warrior, it is Arjuna's *dharma* (duty) to fight. No transgression will result if he does so without attachment to the future consequences of his actions. His soul or spirit will not be contaminated by his deeds. Likewise, *vinyasa* treats the action performed on each breath as ethically neutral and, once completed, disposable. Because *vinyasa* works breath by breath, it is performed with little attachment; the action undertaken on a single breath has little enduring consequence. When it is over, the next breath offers a different experience. Whatever one imagines the result of their actions will be is, at best, approximate. Yogic thought considers such constructs illusory, preventing one from perceiving the actuality. A focus committed to each breath prevents the practitioner from anticipating the future. This is a *vinyasa* interpretation of "yoga is skill in action" (Johnson 2009, 2.50).

Categorisation and the "Spotlight" of Our Attention

In apprehending the material world through the senses, one necessarily engages in a parsing away.[17] The interpretation that is brought about through sensory impressions occurs at the diminution of something else. Such impressions are categorised (or metaphorised). "That smells like a rose – not a gardenia" or "That's as rough as sandpaper – not smooth as glass". This categorisation comes from previous experience – from impressions we have formed of roses or gardenias. But the actual experience of the particular smell; that particular rose; is *that* experience and each experience is unique. The direct encounter with the material world, prior to categorisation, is what is going on in the universe. Categorisation is useful for enhancing appreciation through description, but defining detail is not the same as attempting to experience that which is possible, but which has not become material – *purusha*. When we categorise, the spotlight of our attention focuses on the particular (the smell of that rose and not the gardenia); this "illumination" is generally thought of as consciousness.

Vinyasa describes *purusha* here as having the fundamental nature of always possibly "becoming"; something whose timelessness lies in the fixity of its potentiality. Its permanence is that it is always that which could become, as opposed to *prakriti* – that which "becomes". Though these *vinyasa* definitions might be seen as deviating from the traditional, they have the merits of plausibility and practicality in defining the difference between the realities of material and spiritual. The experience of "unattached action" or the aesthetic emotion of beauty give insight into this *purushic* reality of possibility. *Purusha* and *prakriti* are limitless in their own extraordinary ways. The *Between Space* – the volume of consciousness – is where the causality of *prakriti* engages its operational facility with the potentiality of *purusha* – the place where what is possible is brought into being. Appreciating *purusha* means the acknowledgement of its "becomingness" – before it is given material form and can be categorised. What the *vinyasa* method purports to examine and acknowledge is this indestructible state of potentiality – a beauty that is always latent. Moreover, *vinyasa* considers that the self-consciousness we generally intuit – the ability to categorise or metaphorise – is the name (category) we give to describe ourselves in order to identify what feels to be our personal monad of this "becomingness". *Vinyasa* argues, however, the situation is actually that the self we normally refer to (the spotlight of our attention) is something that has "become" – *prakriti*. The ways in which the terms "self" and "consciousness" are used is confusing for they seem to have two different meanings. There is one generally assumed when referring to awareness of ourselves, particularly when engaged in introspection. In yoga, consciousness is also used to mean "true nature" (Self), wherein one is seen (as is the rest of reality) as *purusha* – not self-aware, but simply in a timeless state of becoming and, as yet, not become.

The "Self"

In both ancient and modern texts, one finds an array of references to the idea that *purusha* is the "essential self" or a "true self". In a popular modern characterisation, *purusha* is "spirit" (and *prakriti* is "matter", hence the Self is not matter). The idea of spirit, however, and what it refers to, is used quite flexibly in yoga circles. In the statement, "I'm a very spiritual person", the sense would not be much changed if the word "soulful" was used instead. The conflation of spirit with soul is misleading: yoga literature is abundant with the idea that souls are capable of transmigration – given to taking up residence temporarily in "matter" bodies. However, the notion of a knowable soul reappearing in subsequent incarnations is contrary to the pursuit of the negation of body and mind to the irreducible – the Self – where there is no mind or consciousness as we experience it in introspection. It is instead a complete self-forgetfulness and merging with the infinite in which there are no traces left of the individual. The potentiality inherent in the "I" or "pure consciousness" that is *purusha* remains unchanged, which the *vinyasi* might argue is intimated in the experience of beauty.

"Matter" seems obvious – it is all that we encounter that has "substance", but we may be misled in this. When we place a hand on a yoga mat, nerve responses are initiated that send electrical signals to various parts of the brain and we rapidly assemble a picture of the mat. Other senses might equally be involved – the olfactory nerves might detect "smell" and they will send electrical stimuli to other parts of the brain; the same with the way our seeing mechanism detects the colour and shape of the mat. The picture assembled by our minds through a multitude of brain functions, however, is not the same as the mat itself. Can we know *prakriti* without this intercession of the senses? The *asana* solution is that to know the mat's "matness", one can approach it through contemplation – to discover its essentiality by looking inward and seeing where one's own essentiality and that of the mat coincide. In so doing, one discovers the essence of all things – something that must have been in us (and all things) all along, but which needed to be *dis-covered* by sifting through and eliminating the accretions of sensual input. In other words, seeing things as they are; not as they appear to be in categorised details. But is this the essentiality (Self) that is meant by *purusha*? And does the savouring of "substance", albeit at a remove, entirely preclude the pursuit of such Self-knowledge?

The appreciation of *prakriti* has been undervalued, as understanding who we are and what we feel and interpret is fascinating. Is it a distraction from the acknowledgement of *purusha*? Only if we believe *prakriti* to be unalterably fixed – that the ways in which we categorise (impressions, thoughts, and interpretations) are final solutions. This scent of this rose is so like every other rose that it is exactly the same. *Vinyasa*, at root, acknowledges the changeability of *prakriti* – interprets and savours it. It accedes that in the *vinyasa* practice nothing is more valuable than anything else – that transitions and postures amount to the same thing; each having their own qualities to savour and interpret. And this may be what is meant by "evenness of mind" (Johnson 2009, 2.48) – a precursor to *purushic* Self-understanding as is *asana's* practice of mind-stilling.

Maya: Illusion or Creativity?

Without being able to say quite what mind or consciousness is, there is agreement on the mechanism it works through. Sensory information is fed by electrical stimuli to various parts of the brain and the motor responses reciprocally activate the body. The imagery that the mind creates (a sensation of burning pain in a muscle; the movement of the leg to stop it – the glorious sight of a tree bathed in summer sun; the memory of a day like it in one's youth that spurs a walk outside) are wholly unique in each individual, as the same experience is construed in different ways. These electrical stimuli are neutral – there are not "burning muscle" electrical stimuli and different "seeing sun" electrical stimuli – but they are construed as such depending on the parts of the brain they reach. In this construing, we find a process of mind that constructs a simulacrum of what is going on and then responds accordingly. Because these constructions are individual and personal, the yoga conception has been that they are *maya* (illusion) or, in an even more extreme reading, that the things the simulacra describe are illusory themselves – appearances of fluctuations of *prakriti* enmeshed in temporality that we – through our mental constructions – accord a mistaken permanence and validity. The yogi, in this theory, assumes that there is an absolute reality (everything that "has been created" or "could be") that these illusions prevent us from accessing.

Maya might be imagined as a path to liberation rather than an impediment to it. One could make participation in *maya* a creative and contributive activity – not merely a receptive misinterpreting. When an artist paints a landscape, they are not pretending it is the same thing as the landscape they depict – it is, prosaically, paint dabbed on canvas. There is no such thing as an objective rendering of the landscape – only the landscape itself can *be* that. It is, instead, a perspective that may give some insight into what absolute reality might actually be; the artist's rendering invites interpretation. Through an aesthetic philosophy each time the yogi executes a posture or performs a sequence, they try to do the same.

VINYASA AS AN AESTHETIC PHILOSOPHY

As presented above, in *vinyasa*, the practitioner behaves like they are a radiance of *pranic* energy that begins at the *mula* and "discharges" up through the torso and out through the legs and beyond to the limit of their volume of consciousness – the *Between Space*. Just as the painter does not mistake his painting for an actual landscape, the *vinyasi* does not believe this to be the way things actually are. It is an imaginative way to engage the multiple parts of body and mind in *dharana/ekagrata* and is a method that, on a breath-by-breath basis, can give additional perspective on how the mind engages with The Absolute in the *Between Space*. There is no attachment to what is perceived, for the next breath brings something new.

The use of art and nature analogies in this chapter endeavours to show a range of possibilities for experiencing yoga as an aesthetic philosophy – it attempts to define the experience of beauty as an entry to the understanding of reality through an appreciation of it. There are other possible and highly creative ways this might be done. Some might be able to evolve techniques based on similar abstractions like trying to see God or love or ethical virtue in all things.

A leitmotif that runs through yogic thought is that "all is suffering". But how would yoga (and religious) *experience* be different if *practice* and *belief* were based on "all is delight"? Suffering or delight seem too categoric or limited for neither permits the beauty of such alloyed notions as a "sweet sadness". There is a difference between yearning and desire. Desire refers to something from which there is separation (I desire chocolate), but which can be satisfied, whereas yearning refers to a kind of separation for which remedy is difficult (yearning for the days of one's youth) and that, however sad it is, also has a "sweetness" attached to it. This idea is one that has informed religions that come from west of the Levant – separation from God, but a yearning to draw nearer. The same could perhaps be said of yoga – its quest for union implies that apparent separateness is a part of what the practice is about. It also may explain why the practices of yoga are meant to be intense. They are motivated by an intense feeling – the sweet sadness of separation. It also suggests that its practices are intensely difficult and must be borne because they will also be intensely rewarding should they work.

Much is made of exposing the Self to ourselves through practising yoga. However, one yogic notion that persists is that the true Self (our "true nature") is the same as *purusha*. In the construct offered above, this would mean that the Self – as is everything in the universe – is also in a state of "becomingness". Whether one can achieve this understanding as a kind of unity through either *asana's* stillness or through *vinyasa's* continual movement is the pursuit of the yogi.

Notes

1 They further argue that, historically, emphasis has swung between the supernatural and the scientific in understanding the interlocked structure of experience/belief/ practice. Most recently, it has swung to such an extent into the scientific that it is unlikely to swing back again. They trenchantly observe: "Attempts to achieve a rapprochement between science and religion are today common, but they inevitably end in adjustments to religious belief, not to scientific findings." (290)

2 Eliade places yoga within the traditions of religious history. He concludes his anthropological treatise on yoga with a summary of where such extrapolations might lead: "He who would attain to comprehension of these 'mysteries' must raise himself to another mode of being, and, to reach it, he must 'die' to this life and sacrifice 'personality' that has issued from temporality, that has been created by history (personality being above all memory of our own history). 'Liberated in life', the *jivan-mukta* no longer possesses a personal consciousness – that is, a consciousness nourished on his own history – but a witnessing consciousness, which is pure lucidity and spontaneity ... (Yoga) finds its place in a universal tradition of the religious history of mankind: the tradition that consists in anticipating death in order to ensure rebirth in a sanctified life – that is, a life made *real* by the incorporation of the sacred." (1958, 363)

3 He also expressed this idea as "all things are requited for fire and fire for all things." Retrieved from Iain McGilchrist, 2009, Notes to Chapter 8: The Ancient World, 58 and 60.

4 Though the concepts of *purusha* and *prakriti* and their relationship are contested in competing (dualistic and monistic) interpretations of Samkhya philosophy, *prakriti* can be understood as "matter", "creation or creativity", or "nature", and *purusha* as

"spirit", "man", "person", "being", or "soul". One popular translation of *purusha* has been "(pure) consciousness" – and sometimes *prakriti* as "consciousness", which is equivocal since the very concept of consciousness is problematic. (Jamal Jones, p.c. 21 October, 2020).

5 *Mulaprakriti* is "primordial", "basic", or "original", while still meaning "that which exists in nature" (Sinha, 1986, 29). *Mulaprakriti* offers a clarification of the classical understanding of the terms in Samkhya philosophy – something that exists (*sat*), cannot originate from non-existence (*asat*). Therefore, it denies the creation of universe and states that universe is unborn and eternal.

6 At the beginning of *Yoga: Immortality and Freedom*, Mircea Eliade introduces four terms, *karma, maya, nirvana*, and *yoga* and gives a description of their significance in the understanding of absolute reality. "(1) The law of universal causality, which connects man with the cosmos and condemns him to transmigrate indefinitely. This is the law of *karma*. (2) The mysterious process that engenders and maintains the cosmos and, in so doing, makes possible the 'eternal return' of existences. This *māyā*, cosmic illusion, endured (even worse – accorded validity) by man as long as he is blinded by ignorance (*avidya*). (3) Absolute reality, 'situated' somewhere beyond the cosmic illusion woven by *māyā* and beyond human experience as conditioned by *karma*; pure Being, the Absolute, by whatever name it may be called --the Self (*ātman*), *Brahman*, the unconditioned, the transcendent, the immortal, the indestructible, *nirvāna*, etc. (4) The means of attaining to Being, the effectual techniques for gaining liberation. This corpus of means constitutes Yoga properly speaking.", 3.

7 The terms for the idea of "great unity" abound. Totality, oneness, absolute, apeiron, absolute reality, cosmos, macrocosm, universe, reality, the whole, *Brahman*, the All. These terms endeavour to express the concept of "that which is all" and each has a slightly different nuance. Throughout, we have used a number of these in the hope that the various shades of meaning might be accommodated.

8 Jason Birch "The Proliferation of Asana-s in Late-Medieval Yoga Texts", in *Yoga and Transformation Historical and Contemporary Perspectives*, edited by Karl Baier, Philipp A. Maas, and Karin Preisendanz. (Vienna: Vienna University Press, 2018), 101–180. In his work on the proliferation and source material of *asana*, Jason Birch states: "As far as I am aware, the prominent modern practices of suryanamaskara and vinyasa are absent in medieval yoga texts." Birch further notes: "In his biography of his teacher Krsnamacarya, A. G. Mohan ... defines vinyasa and states his belief that vinyasa was Krsnamacarya's innovation: 'A special feature of the asana system of Krishnamacharya was vinyasa. Many yoga students are no doubt familiar with this word – it is increasingly used now, often to describe the "style" of a yoga class, as in "hatha vinyasa" or "vinyasa flow". Vinyasa is essential, and probably unique, to Krishnamacharya's teachings. As far as I know, he was the first yoga master in the last century to introduce the idea. A vinyasa, in essence, consists of moving from one asana, or body position, to another, combining breathing with the movement.'" 138–139.

9   Martin Rees' very readable book gives a clear idea of the scale and composition of
     the universe.

10   The idea of *yama* as a restraint might also be linked to Yama the god of death: the
     idea of death, or cessation, could be equated with the idea in breath retentions
     where the discharge of *prana* is meant to be stopped or held inert. Swami Rama
     suggests, however, that it is *ayama* that would mean "expansion or manifestation".
     (Rama, 1979, 72).

11   The author has encountered the term in Malayasia as "point of origin" and, in
     back translations of Malay to English on glosbe.com such definitions as beginning,
     cause, origin, original, and parent are found. This is not surprising as Indian civil-
     isation and religion began in the seventh century to exert influence on the Ancient
     Malay language.

12   Sinha (1986) suggests that while Patanjali describes *pratayahara* in 2:54–55 of the
     Yoga Sutras, that the decisive description is found in 2:33, 53.

13   The immensity of the visible universe (a size of 10–14 billion light years) is some-
     thing we represent as a number, but which has no practical bearing on the way
     most of us live our lives. When we begin to scope out how long it took the first
     Voyager spacecraft (launched 1977) to reach the place where our sun's atmos-
     phere runs into interstellar winds – nearly 30 years – and when we realise that
     signals from these spacecrafts travelling at the speed of light take around 15 hours
     to reach us and that the next nearest star is something close to 4.5 light years
     away, we are already close to the limit of practical imagining. To then consider
     that our sun is just one of approximately 100 billion stars in our galaxy and that
     within the range of our telescopes there exists at least that many galaxies, we are
     in the realm of perplexing immensity. And the very small is just as bewildering.
     Discussing both the concepts of size and the scale of time in the very early for-
     mation of the universe, Martin Rees elegantly writes, "An absolute limit to any
     credible backward extrapolation is set by quantum theory. The key concept of this
     theory is Heisenberg's uncertainty relation, which tells us that the more accurately
     you want to locate or localise something, the more energetic are the quanta – the
     packets of energy – you need. There is a limit when the energy is so concentrated
     that it risks imploding into a black hole. This limit is the Planck Length: its value is
     10^{-33} cm – smaller than a proton by about 19 powers of 10. This minuscule length,
     divided by the speed of light, defines the smallest measurable time interval, the
     Planck Time, about 10^{-44} seconds." (Rees 2001, 127).

14   Theoretically, the volume of consciousness could be infinite (boundless like the
     apeiron), but, to limit it somewhat, one could say it might be around 14 billion
     light years in every direction because that would be the confinement of the uni-
     verse as set by the limits of the speed of light and the assumed rate of expansion of
     the universe. It could also be assumed that everything beyond that limit is also like
     what the limits of sense can apprehend.

15   *Samadhi* "completion or accomplishment", "intense or ultimate contemplation", "final resting placing (or tomb)" (Jones, p.c. 21 October, 2020).

16   The expression "leap of faith" is particularly associated with the Danish philosopher Søren Kierkegaard. He contended that the premise underlying faith was that it was unproveable. His personal "leap of faith" was a religious one, but he also articulated the idea that there were moral (what is good and bad) and aesthetic (what is deemed beautiful) "leaps of faith". Importantly, he saw faith as a lived experience.

17   A debt is owed to Iain McGilchrist's extraordinary book, *The Master and His Emissary*, (on brain lateralisation) for his cogent consideration of categorisation as well as his thoughts on the role of melancholy – and Jorge Luis Borges from whom he borrowed the apt title).

Appendix 1: Reflection and Experimentation

1.1 PHYSICAL PHILOSOPHY

Philosophy seeks to examine difficult questions to understand the complexity of existence. Broadly, philosophy considers the subjects of ethics (good and bad), epistemology (knowledge), aesthetics (conceptions of beauty), metaphysics (time, space, God), and politics. Philosophers "think" to clarify questions and to provide evidence for explanations. In teaching, do you feel it is possible to teach yoga without a philosophic dimension? If so, how is it distinguished from other forms of athletic practice?

1.2 EVENNESS OR STILLNESS

One of the metaphysical tenets of yoga is that there is a state of "pure consciousness", which is a self-less, unchanging, indestructible, and eternal state of existence. Is it even possible to ponder a "self-less" primordial existence since we can only know this existence through our minds (embodied experience)? What are the possibilities for philosophical discovery through physical practice? Does evenness of breath, coupled with evenness of movement, result in evenness of mind; and is this mental evenness a prerequisite for the yogic inquiry into the nature of the universe? Does lack of movement and absence of breath still the mind; and does this serve to reveal the nature of pure consciousness? Do any of these premises inform your practice? If so, how? Do you feel that your individual experience of these methods gives you authority to convincingly teach?

1.3 BROACHING THE INFINITE

Many terms are used to suggest the whole of reality. For instance, Hegel (Herbermann 1913) used *The Absolute* to refer to "the sum of all being, actual and potential." Other terms that are similarly used might include Totality, *Brahman*, The All, Reality, Apeiron, Cosmos, Great Unity, etc. Such concepts, in both philosophy and yoga, require feats of extraordinary imagining, but it is not "anything goes". The scale of physical reality is vast – it could be infinite and boundless, or it might be something that is presumed 250 times the size we can observe (based on the way light behaves as it moves through the curvature of space) – and yet both philosophy and yoga attempt to confront this by studying what they can and theorising from what they infer. This exercise is meant to draw one's attention to the magnitude of this scale. In this case, the paradox of disciplined and structured imagining of hypotheticals facilitates coherent results for studying the boundless. How might you imagine the immensity of the universe and how through a physical practice can you engage with this?

Analogy is one way to do this imagining. Place an object in front of you and place a second object one inch away from the first. This is meant to represent the distance from the Earth to the moon. The distance from the Earth to the sun is approximately 93 million miles. Light takes eight-and-a-half minutes to travel this distance. With the moon to Earth ratio above, that would place the sun about ten yards distant; perhaps the furthest wall away from you if you are in a room. The edge of the solar system is called the Heliopause and is reckoned to be around 11.3 billion miles away from the sun. This might be something like the distance to your nearest shopping centre. From here to the nearest star is about 4.3 light years or, by the one inch to the moon scale, about 470 miles. The distance from where you are to the centre of our galaxy is about 18,000 light years. On our scale, this works out to approximately 200,000 miles – close to driving your car to the moon, which, if you drove at 60 miles per hour for 24 hours per day, would take around four months to do. The distance to the edge of the perceivable universe is around 14 billion light years. That would take 238,000 years of driving.

If the room you are in or the vistas you can see are your perceivable universe, how do you practice in a way that surpasses the perception of your senses?

1.4 TIME, SPACE, AND THE VOLUME OF CONSCIOUSNESS

What do the senses tell us about space? The size of the volume of consciousness is something accessed through the reciprocal relationship of the senses and our motor responses. The arena of these interactions is an imagined place outside of our physical bodies where our actions and that which appears to be "other" co-mingle. Most physical practice is self-referential – detecting such things as the stresses of muscular stretch, stability of balance, or joint movement and their effects on consciousness. However, *vinyasa* practice suggests that the world in which the body moves is equally important and influential for the understanding of self and our construction of reality.

When we place our hands on the floor, they detect comparatively obvious information about its texture, its evenness, or its stability, but also about the density (Is it wood? Concrete? Rubber mat?) and something so obvious it may be overlooked – the effect of gravity. The awareness of gravity shows that there are forces and substances beyond the immediate contact between hand and floor. This implies the existence of a space greater than what can easily be perceived. Other senses inform us about the space too. Smells give information about who else may be in the room or incense may indicate a ritual space. The reverberation of sound off of walls, the subtle taste of the air we breathe, and, of course, the eyes tell us spatial information that our consciousness interprets. How might you investigate the way you interpret the relationship between time and space?

Drag your fingertips along a table. Drag your fingertips along the table as slowly as you can. Drag your fingertips along the table as slowly as you can and exhale through the nose at a speed that exactly matches the speed of your fingertips. Try it on an inhale. What differences do you notice? Perform a Sun Salute attempting the above with the fingertips and evaluate the sensation of the fingertips as they move through the air and when they are planted on the ground. Can you sustain the evenness of the breath throughout? How do these efforts affect your mental processes? What are the differences between the way the fingertips relate to the solidity of the table or mat and the way they relate to what is sensed when they move through the air? How would you characterise the differences between what you impart to the table or mat and what you impart to the air? Take an inhale and, holding the breath, perform the entirety of a Sun Salute. How does this change the evenness of the movement? How does this change the sensations? Do you value what you experience more or less (or just the same) when you do actions in a fast or a slow way and why?

1.5 ELIMINATING THE SUPERFLUOUS; IDENTIFYING THE ESSENTIAL

If the "truth" of reality lies in discovering what is essential and what is superfluous, what could you dispense with? *Vinyasa* has one solution – a melding with all that is other through aesthetic emotion so that essentiality is experienced through a unity of a multitude of factors. *Asana* attempts a reduction of engagement of the embodied self until only the essence of "pure consciousness" remains. In both these methods, what is necessary (focus, strength, stamina, or simplicity)? What is superfluous (worry, ambition, relationships, fear, or desire)? If you take away such things as these, do you take away or enhance "appreciation" and "discrimination"?

When the superfluous is surrendered are you able to experience a "bliss" or "serenity" or "awe" that was made unavailable by these "attachments"? Or are these contrasts necessary for bliss or suffering to be experienced? If bliss is eternal, can one appreciate it without the contrast of suffering? Do attachments necessarily cause suffering or act as impediments to bliss? Are you willing to "not take pleasure" in all that exists now in order to experience the ultimate bliss of nonattachment? Are you convinced that ultimate bliss is attainable through physical practice? If not, how does this impact on your practice and your teaching?

1.6 AESTHETIC PHILOSOPHY: LEARNING TO SEE

How does a person refine their aesthetic appreciation of yoga? This exercise is about considering and realising the qualitative aspects of improving one's aesthetic experience (rather than skill in imitation) and understanding that meaning evolves during the process of execution. Randomly choose a yoga photograph. Study the photograph for things you might not have wholly appreciated at first glance. What are the elements of the background? Is it in a gym, photography studio, or outdoors? What paraphernalia are around, are there other people and what are they doing? How is it lit? What do you think happened right before the photograph? What happened right after? If you can see the face of the subject, what are their eyes doing? What are their lips doing? How about their hands and feet? Can you imitate these and, if so, what do you feel when you do it? Take a picture of your face (hands or feet) doing the same thing. In evaluating the picture of yourself, consider two things: how would you go about making it better resemble the original and how might you simply retake the picture to make yourself look better in your estimation. You have to actually DO it, rather than think about it.

Choose or imagine a posture or a sequence. What would be the ideal setting (a studio, beach, mountaintop, a city street) to do such movements? The ideal apparel? With eyes shut or open? Focus inward or outward? What music could accompany it? Does it look heavy or light? What would you need to prepare to bring these out of potentiality and into being?

1.7 HOW DO WE UNDERSTAND SOMETHING AS EPHEMERAL AS *PURUSHA*?

If *purusha* is potentiality, how can you begin to examine this potentiality in physical practice? Can you bring something into existence that is possible, but not yet realised? There are structural aspects of each of our bodies that make us capable of certain things (splits) and not necessarily of others (straddle splits). What is it fruitful for you to bring into being and why? Does this bring insight into *purusha*? Or is its value limited to *prakriti*?

References

Bhaktivedanta Narayana Gosvami Maharaja, Sri Srimad and Śrīla Bhaktivinoda Ṭhākura, *Pure Bhakti: Bhajana-rahasya*, 2nd Edition. New Delhi: Gaudiya Vedanta Publications, 2015.

Birch, Jason. "The proliferation of asana-s in late-medieval yoga texts." In *Yoga and transformation historical and contemporary perspectives*, edited by Karl Baier, Philipp A. Maas, and Karin Preisendanz, 101–180. Vienna: Vienna University Press, 2018.

Coomaraswamy, Ananda K. *The dance of Siva: essays on Indian art and culture.* New York: Dover, 1985.

Cooper, David E. "Introduction." In *Aesthetics: the classic readings*, edited by David E. Cooper, 1–10. Oxford: Blackwell Publishers, 1997.

Eliade, Mircea. *Yoga immortality and freedom*, translated by Willard R. Trask. Princeton: Bollingen Foundation, Princeton University Press, 1958.

Herbermann, Charles, ed. "The Absolute." In *Catholic Encyclopedia*. New York: Robert Appleton Company, 1913.

Jakubczak, Marzenna. "The purpose of non-theistic devotion in the classical Indian tradition of Sāmkhya-Yoga." *Argument*, vol. 4 (January, 2014): 55–68.

Jaspers, Karl. *The origin and goal of history*, translated by Michael Bullock. London: Routledge, 1955.

Johnson, Williams J., translator. *The Bhagavad Gita*. Oxford: Oxford University Press, 2009.

Lewis-Williams, David and David Pearce. *Inside the neolithic mind*. London: Thames and Hudson, 2005.

Mallinson, James and Mark Singleton. *Roots of yoga*. New York: Penguin Books, 2017.

McGilchrist, Iain. *The master and his emissary: the divided brain and the making of the Western world*. New Haven: Yale, 2009.

Rama, Swami. *The science of breath*. Delhi: The Himalayan Institute Press, 1979.

Rama, Swami. *Sacred journey: living purposefully and dying gracefully*. Delhi: Himalayan Institute Hospital Trust, 2002.

Rees, Martin. *Our cosmic habitat*. Princeton: Princeton University Press, 2001.

Sinh, Pancham. *The Hatha Yoga Pradipika: Sanskrit text with English translation*. New Delhi: Munshiram Manoharlal Publishers, 1915.

Sinha, Phulgenda. *The Gita as it was: rediscovering the original Bhagavad Gita*. LaSalle: Open Court, 1986.

Stark, Rodney and William Sims Bainbridge. *The future of religion*. Berkeley: University of California Press, 1985.

Tarnas, Richard. *The passion of the Western mind: understanding the ideas that have shaped our world view*. London: Pimlico, 1991.

Vasu, Rai Bahadur Srisa Chandra, translators. *Siva Samhita*. New Delhi: Munshiram Manoharlal Publishers, 1914–15.

Chapter Two
Teaching Yoga
Methodology, Meaning, and Ritual

One of the most powerful aspects of drumming and the reason people have done it since the beginning of being human is that it changes people's consciousness. Through rhythmic repetition of ritual sounds, the body, the brain and the nervous system are energized and transformed. When a group of people play a rhythm for an extended period of time, their brain waves become entrained to the rhythm and they have a shared brain wave state. The longer the drumming goes on, the more powerful the entrainment becomes. It's really the oldest holy communion.

Layne Redmond[1]

METHODS FOR MODERN YOGA: THE POTENTIAL IN RITUAL

To sustain a clear philosophy (theory), one must devise a method by which philosophical precepts can be put to the test. The method should provide a vehicle for experimentation – a proving ground for one's theory – and generate a number of techniques that can be used to carry out investigations. If the *theory, method,* and *techniques* are cohesive, they may be applied to any *form*. The form (the yoga postures and movements one actually practices) is inconsequential, since its manner of practice will

DOI: 10.4324/9781003181910-3

be executed through techniques, that are informed by the method which is soundly based in theory. Simply, the practice will always be in service of experimentation grounded in intellectual rigour.[2]

There are many methods in the teaching of physical yoga that encourage experiential learning. The analysis that follows will look at some of the ways that practice, when executed through focused and cohesive teaching methods, may be understood as a transformational pedagogy. Yoga practitioners may seek personal transformation in an effort to better understand the nature of reality. Therefore, this chapter begins by looking at acts of transformation (rituals) through the disciplines of performance theory, psychology, and anthropology. Rituals are used by all cultures to assist members through significant transitions and are the principal site of ecstatic (intense) experience, meaning making, and innovation for both individuals and the group that enacts them.

YOGA: RITUAL OF TRANSFORMATION

> The sacred is not in heaven or far away. It is all around us, and small
> human rituals can connect us to its presence.
>
> Alma Luz Villanueva[3]

To understand the transformational process, it is necessary to briefly explore the concept of ritual in the anthropological literature. For most, rituals are only understood in the context of religious enactment. But rituals occur in all aspects of life, often to fully mundane ends. Rituals will be prevalent wherever the outcome of a desired task is uncertain. Sporting events, for example, are rife with ritualistic behaviours, which are exacerbated by the increasing pressure (stress) of performance. In baseball, players up at bat have elaborate rituals, as do the pitchers who oppose them. This is understandable when one concedes the difficulty of getting on base for the batter or throwing a strikeout for the pitcher. Having greater control over the outcome, those in the outfield show little to no ritualistic behaviour as they eye a ball they are about to catch. Why does the batter go through a series of routinised gestures? Because they believe that performing these will increase their chance of success or, more properly, not performing them will risk failure. The gestures in this sense are magical. They are able to enlist the aid of supernatural forces for the mundane ends of hitting a homerun. Similarly, because the ultimate goal of yoga is enlightenment, the outcome is far from certain.

It should be no surprise that ritual behaviour should accompany these lofty aspirations. The redundancy of Sun Salutations practiced repeatedly along with chanting (either call and response or through repetition), set sequences practiced daily, the repetition of daily practice itself, all illustrate ritualistic action.

Rituals may be described as any behaviour characterised by *repetition*, *redundancy*, and *stylisation*. Rituals, however practiced, are never gratuitous, but are purposeful, and therefore carry considerable meaning. In *Rites of Passage*, Arnold van Gennep identifies rituals as having three stages: *separation*, *transition*, and *incorporation* (van Gennep, 1960).[4] In the first stage – separation – initiates remove themselves (or are removed) from their quotidian and mundane status. This leads to the second stage – transition – during which initiates attempt the process of transformation. The stage of transition is potentially dangerous or disruptive because the experience may lead to mental or bodily harm, perhaps even death. It is, however, "safe" in the sense that initiates are free from social and cultural condemnation (van Gennep, 1960, "The Territorial Passage", 15–25). Transition is a "time out of time" where cultural and social norms may be examined (tested and/or affirmed), and where normal rules of understanding are suspended. This contestation often leads to innovation, since, in the ritual context, boundaries may be "safely" tested. In the final stage – incorporation – initiates are reinstated into the social order in a transformed state.

Transition is often characterised by an experience of catharsis or of altered states of consciousness. While rules are suspended, and people act outside of cultural constraints, much can go wrong. This *liminality* (borderline status) threatens successful incorporation but allows for exploration and experimentation (creativity). Liminality also may lead to conflict since the suspension of rules allows for all things to be contested, even those outside of the ritual context. Clifford Geertz refers to this same process and the creative potential in transformation as "deep play." (Geertz 2005). Johan Huizinga, in his 1938 publication, *Homo Ludens* ('Man the Player'), speaks of a "magic circle" to metaphorically circumscribe the ritual space as a "time out of time" (see Figure 2.1). This magic circle is characterised as a "sacred space" in which actions occur. Within this space, actions are regulated by different rules and when performed are attributed different (symbolic) meaning. The actions which take place within this magic circle may both test and reaffirm cultural norms, for in this space, where normal rules are

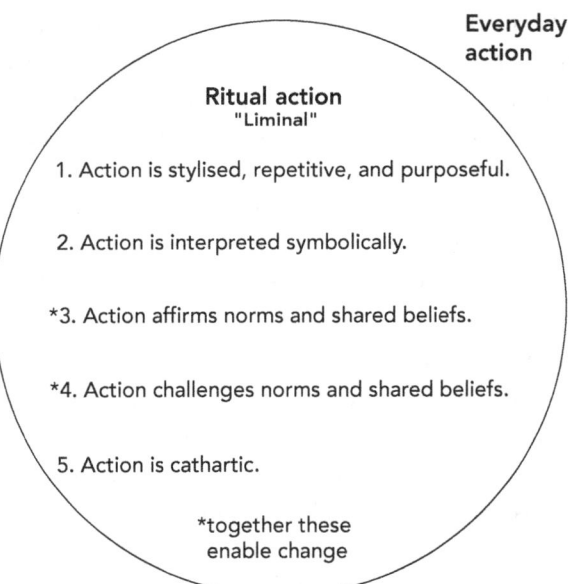

Figure 2.1 The Magic Circle: A graphic representation of ritual

suspended, creativity is possible. The experiences therein often result in catharsis (Huizinga 2016).

Yoga may be seen as a ritual practice. There is an expectation that, although gathering in a group class, silence will be observed or that conversations are held at a whisper. One goes barefoot into the practice space, clothing may be revealing or form fitting, and men may even practice bare-chested. The teacher may touch students' bodies, often in places that are considered off limits to anyone but intimates, and breathing is synchronised and audible. Such actions have different meaning in the yoga studio than they would performed just outside its doors, signalling that their interpretation is mediated by a ritual context. The realms of art, sport, and religion were all seen as occurring within the magic circle according to Huizinga. It is the "frame" that makes the event sacred and the meaning symbolic. Likewise, with physical yoga practice, one should be careful not to judge the meaning of actions simply by their performance. It is the liminality created in this context that allows for transformation. Victor Turner has described liminality as the mother of invention (Turner 1967). One can see the important and powerful role that ritual plays in the process of change within the context of teaching yoga. The yoga teacher has the opportunity to initiate and guide the progression of a ritual, allowing students to have a deeper experience in somatic practice.

Thomas Driver argues that the techniques of ritual appeal to "laws" that are culturally specific, unlike the perception we have of invariant laws found in things we designate as "science." "Magic," therefore, the transformative power of ritual action, "operates within socio-cultural frameworks of reality" (Driver 2006, 172). The transformative power of yoga is possible within the context of the shared rules and meanings of the "yoga community". These rules do not have to follow the laws of science or larger society and the beliefs that support them can be held simultaneously with a separate set of cultural beliefs. Therefore, the modern yoga teacher may live in the world and likewise be apart from it, in an environment they create in order to allow for the possibility of ecstatic experience. Rituals, because they operate in a context that lies outside of the social rules and structures of mundane reality, allow practitioners to have an experience that might not be possible in their socially constrained everyday lives. If you do not suspend the norms, you cannot both affirm and/or contest them – the outcome of any ritual enactment. The yoga teacher's and students' adoption of this separate set of beliefs for the purpose of ritual experimentation in yoga is highly productive when understood in the symbolic context. Such beliefs are working hypotheses and should not be presented as literal truths supported by facts (as with scientific truths) lest they lose their transformative potential.

The arts are "sacred" (categorically, like ritual) because they are interpreted through a different set of rules. Normal modes of interpretation are suspended. Symbolic interpretation is required (rather than a utilitarian one). This allows for fluidity of interpretation as well as different individual experiences, since the rules for interpretation are more flexible. Part of ritual is to engender an aesthetic reaction, where the intention of the creator has coherence with its execution (intentions are realised in form and movement in yoga). The yoga teacher instructs the student how to be both the doer and the observer. Students learn how to critically observe their own aesthetic creation. To be effective as a ritual, yoga classes need clarity of purpose. This clarity is the responsibility of the teacher, who acts as ritual specialist, guiding initiates through the process (ritual stages of practice), articulating and focusing on clear goals, keeping initiates safe, contextualising their experience, and debriefing them as the ritual ends.

The Characteristics of Ritual Action

From the perspective of anthropology and performance theory, Richard Schechner (1985) proposes features of ritual action that may help to elucidate the ritual nature of yoga practice (Schechner 2008/2009).[5] The following eight *characteristics* are found in yoga practice and, once recognised, can be used by teachers to enhance meaningful experience and create heightened awareness for yoga students:

BEHAVIOURS/ACTIONS CHANGE THEIR FUNCTION

For example, in yoga practice, breathing is no longer an autonomic function, but is controlled (through slowing and synchronisation) to move life force (*prana*) and provide focus. Physical contortions are ways to "lose the body", and directed observation (meditation) is a vehicle for spiritual evolution. The use of objects also takes on new meanings. The use, placement, and spacing of the practice mat, the gathering and arranging of props, and the positioning of icons and images, all have specific, symbolic, and venerated meaning. Because they are more than utilitarian, they are to be kept clean and well cared for.

Cultural taboos are often violated as a result of this ritual context. Bare feet are seen as clean, rather than polluting. In some systems, one is even expected to kiss the guru's feet and bow down before them, practices which are in violation of Western values and behaviours.[6] The consumption of water may be discouraged, as it dulls the fire of *tapas* (ritual heat). Audible breathing, public "sleeping" (*savasana*), and sitting on the floor are desirable behaviours, if not required of participants. In some systems, one is expected to perform rigorous physical work without sweating. In Ashtanga (Jois) Yoga, if one does sweat, it should be massaged back into the skin (Jois 2010).[7] These unconventional behaviours are all illustrative of a ritually defined context.

THE RITUALIZED MOVEMENT BECOMES INDEPENDENT OF ITS ORIGINAL MOTIVATION AND DEVELOPS ITS OWN MOTIVATING MECHANISMS

The movements and shapes executed in yoga appear random but may be defined as a "sacred geometry" (Iyengar), or perfectly sequenced for spiritual and/or physical progression (Ashtanga and Bikram). Students may progress only at the direction of their teacher (Ashtanga) or practice certain movements at certain times of the day or in response to seasonal, psychological, or astronomical conditions (Ayurveda[8] or Ashtanga Moon Days[9]). Stillness and movement are used for specific purposes unique to yoga practice. Alchemical powers may be unleashed by performing certain postures: Peacock Pose may make you immune to snakebites, Lion Pose may give you strength, and splits may connect you to the mythical qualities of the avatar, Hanuman.

MOVEMENTS ARE EXAGGERATED AND RHYTHMIC

Repetition and stylisation of movements are epitomised in Sun Salutations, but also may be seen in the holding of postures for five breaths in Ashtanga, or the 60- and 30-second holds of each repeated posture in Bikram. The effort to perform extreme bodily contortions and deeper back bends or splits are other examples. Breath is rhythmically controlled through metre, interruption, and ratio, and breath is both lengthened and often held for long periods of time on both the inhale and the exhale.

Movements and shapes may also be exaggerated to the point of discomfort, wherein the practitioner is expected to "push through"; deliberately concealing pain or causing injury in an effort to seek equanimity in difficult circumstances or push past "blockages" (to mind, spirit, emotion, body) attributed to the ego. Symmetry or asymmetry are often practiced ritualistically. In most traditions evolving from Krishnamacharya, for example, postures are performed on both sides, but always first on the right.[10] Practicality is not the stuff of ritual meaning.

MOVEMENTS FREQUENTLY FREEZE INTO POSTURES

Many systems in yoga are characterised by repetitive movements punctuated by holding. Ashtanga Vinyasa is the classic example of such a system, although it can also be seen in Sivananda Yoga derivatives as in the act of intermittent breath holding (*kumbaka*) in *pranayama* practices. In particular, *nadi shodana* and *khaplabhati* are patterned with intermittent movement and holding.

THRESHOLDS FOR EXPRESSING THE BEHAVIOUR ARE LOWERED

Rules for ritual expression, once learned, may be communicated through small indications of larger processes. The greeting *"namaste"*, for example, invokes a connectedness between energetic bodies, which may not yet be experienced in action. Saying that one is "already perfect as they are" insinuates that any effort will be a legitimately meaningful effort – an expression of culturally shared beliefs. Simply chanting *Om* signals a communion with the universe and the powers of creation. The final pose, *savasana*, is a symbolic death and may even be considered practice for the merging that occurs at one's actual death.

SEVERAL MOVEMENTS ARE COMPRESSED INTO STEREOTYPED, SIMPLER MOVEMENTS

Simplification is found in the many traditional movement transitions in yoga and other ritualised activities. There is an infinite number of ways to go from sitting to standing, but these options are reduced and simplified in yoga transitions. Routinisation of movements leads to stereotypical sequences, like those associated with getting into and out of *savasana*,[11] adding to the ritual force of the movement.

BEHAVIOUR AS SIGNAL BECOMES UNAMBIGUOUS

Behaviours are given specific meanings in the context of the studio or practice space. One is expected to obey the teacher's commands, unless one is given the option to choose their own modifications. Speaking amongst students is generally discouraged in practice spaces. In alignment with studio norms, applause for accomplishments may be encouraged as a way to strongly express support and affirmation for others. The chanting of *Om* may be used to signal clearly either the beginning or end of the ritual process. The same is true of the posture *savasana*. The greeting of *namaste* may be expected of practitioners, much like the Catholic exchange "may peace be with you, and with you," to signal community membership and hopes for serenity.

THE SPATIAL ORIENTATION OF THE BEHAVIOUR CHANGES FROM ITS ORDINARY OCCURRENCE

The parallels to physical yoga practice are not difficult to assess here. Special meaning is given to one's orientation in space; students are instructed to place their mats in certain configurations with specific spacing. In both Bikram and Ashtanga systems, teachers may place more advanced students in the front of the practice space. In other systems, students may face one another; this orientation meant to enhance the shared nature of the practice experience. The touching that occurs in yoga classes either between teacher and student in assisting and adjusting, or between students in partner postures or other acts of communion (holding hands, staring in each other's eyes, etc.) are in violation of normal boundaries that regulate physical contact.[12]

These eight characteristics illustrate how teachers who understand the potential power of ritual enactment are able to create deeper, more meaningful, and potentially transformational experiences for their students. To best utilise ritual action as a tool, one must also understand that a yoga class is a ritual progression. The teacher's direction of this progression provides a method for structuring classes that is more likely to lead to cathartic experience.

THE RITUAL PROGRESSION OF PRACTICE

As noted, according to van Gennep, rituals progress through three phases each marking a stage of transformation. A *Rite of Passage* is a ritual that marks an individual leaving one group or state to enter another. It involves a significant change of status within the social or cultural context. Similarly, van Gennep distinguished a *Rite of Intensification*, as a change in status, not by the individual, but by the group. Both rituals are important transitions that are recognised by members of a group. A yoga class may function as a Rite of Passage (for each individual), a Rite of Intensification (for the group), or simultaneously both (van Gennep 1960, "Individuals and Groups", 26–40). In a yoga class, although each individual may begin their ritual experience (*separation*) at different times, there is a moment when everyone becomes formally engaged in the ritual process. The chanting of *Om* at the beginning of a class is such a moment of coming together. As the progression continues, students may experience *transition* together as they simultaneously move through Sun Salutations, and later *incorporation* in the shared silence of *savasana*.

Separation readies one to enter the ritual "play" where the actual change may occur. The word *play* is used here in the way Huizinga has defined it; it is a fundamental aspect and generator of culture. Play is behaviour that is full of symbolic meaning – it is not frivolous as the term may suggest – and is enacted in the realm of ritual, in contrast to *work*, which is mundane behaviour enacted for utilitarian ends. The cultural meaning of "work" is obvious and apparent, but the meaning of "play" is nuanced and open to a range of interpretations, which may lead to creative expression or innovation (Huizinga 2016). One may, for example, drink a sip of wine as a pairing with food because one is thirsty (work), but drinking a sip of wine in communion has symbolic meaning that is only understood by those who have knowledge of this Catholic ritual practice (play). The meaning cannot be known simply through an observation of the actions taking place. Without context and shared cultural knowledge, actions are given meaning based on their everyday functions.

The Stage of Separation

In the stage of *separation*, the initiate is removed from their original status, one that is characterised by their life in the mundane world of work, family, and social relations.

In a yoga class, separation may be signalled simply (ringing a bell, chanting *Om*, placing hands in prayer, setting an intention) or through a complex set of procedures. For individuals, the commencement and duration of the separation stage may be experienced uniquely. For some, the separation commences in the class itself, for others it may begin when they dress for class, and for others still, it may accompany the removal of their socks and the placement of their mat. Rites of Intensification are generally more exacting in their stages, as the group must pass through each stage together. It is during this period that initiates will recognise the leaving of their mundane status and agree to embark on an experience of transition together. This stage may be lengthy or attenuated, depending on the difficulty of the transition.

Separation may start at various locations – when leaving work to go to class (forsaking daily stressors), when changing into yoga clothing (ritual garments), or when entering the studio door (ritual space). There are many symbolic indicators that ease this transition: incense may be burning, iconography may adorn the space, the lights may be dimmed, people may be whispering. At the door to the studio, shoes will be taken off and unnecessary items will be placed in special compartments. Students enter the space barefoot, and place their mats in an appropriate position, oriented according to the customs of the studio. At the front of the space is an altar, which indicates the focal point for the ritual of practice. Each studio has its own unique rules for decorum and behaviour, but some socialising is usually permitted before the next stage of the ritual begins. This socialising is generally subdued as students acknowledge that separation has begun and soon the class will start as well. Some may take to their mats and practice solitary, "warming up" (mini rituals) of their own, either stretching, breathing, or meditating. Soon, the teacher either enters and greets the students, or indicates that the class is about to begin, by dimming the lights, adjusting the music, and greeting the students with ritual language (Sanskrit).

The Stage of Transition

As the class begins, students are moved into the next stage of the ritual – *transition*. Transition is what most think of as "ritual"; the stage where the majority of the duration and elaboration of action occurs. Each aspirant's progression will be measured by how well they execute the challenges presented in practice. In a class or training, students are taken through a series of experiences that provide the opportunity for learning through both the reification and questioning of their beliefs about the world and their place in it. Yoga utilises somatic principles to bring students to this place of exploration, albeit within a set of rules (theory) for interpretation of these experiences. An effective transition is coherent in its structure and sequenced in a way to maximise the possibility of change. The successful commencement of this transition (the class itself) is of special importance for the yoga teacher, since it will determine whether students successfully enter the ritual and potential process of transformation. The use of ritual as a powerful device for successfully guiding students through experiences of discovery and the responsibility that accompanies a teacher's role as ritual specialist in creating or enhancing meaning should not be underestimated. The status of the student or trainee may change during a ritual progression, but the status of the teacher or trainer does not. The ritual operator does not go through the ritual because they must remain aloof so as to guide it.

In yoga, although methods may vary, techniques like breath control, attention to breathing, physical engagement, mental focus, and manipulations of proprioception in stillness and movement are employed to achieve a heightened state of embodiment, and thereby deeper sensory experience. The possibility of catharsis is based on the legitimacy of this heightened sensorial experience consistent with the aspirants' cultural reality. Teachers may inadvertently create "empty" rituals. A teacher trainer, for example, may use the cultural artefacts of Indian and other

Eastern cultures (the giving of Sanskrit names, the wearing of garb or mala beads, the playing of singing bowls) in an attempt to create a meaningful ritual and mark the transformation. However, if these symbols lack cultural authenticity for the aspirant, the ritual may only serve to extend the "liminality" of the experience – the playfulness and unreality – rather than permanently and significantly leading to a change in status.[13]

As Eliade termed it, *enstacy* is the experience of ecstatic catharsis, generated through an aspirant's own (internal) efforts. He proposed that this internal mystical experience (a direct connection with divinity) is what separated yoga from similar experiences in Western traditions, which relied on a religious specialist as an intermediary.[14] A yoga teacher has the potential to facilitate mystical experience, although this change is generally incremental in the modern studio setting. The success of any ritual depends on the collaboration between the ritual specialist (the teacher in this instance) and the aspirant, which produces a genuine change that can be plausibly maintained once the ritual has ended.

The Stage of Incorporation

Transition usually concludes with the final posture, *savasana*, although specific traditions may have "finishing sequences" that signal the nearing of the conclusion of practice. This may include *pranayama*, inversions, final postures (supine twists and backbends are quite common). *Savasana* is an overt symbol of ritual transformation; where a student "dies" (in Corpse Pose), ending the period of ritual testing. The final stage of the ritual progression is *incorporation*. Here the student is "reborn" in a new status, one in which they may be more or less transformed. As with the beginning, the conclusion of the ritual (transition) is of special concern for the teacher, since the effectiveness of this stage will determine the successful integration of the transformation obtained during the ritual process. The teacher's role as facilitator is important but limited, since the individual experience of transition will determine the status into which the student emerges once awoken from Corpse Pose. The entrance into the stage of incorporation is often marked by a sacred sound (singing bowl, tingsha, or bell). Generally, the student is asked to move into foetal position (symbolic of their emergence) and to come up to sitting with eyes closed (like a newborn). The class may end with chanting or the greeting *"namaste"*, which is an acknowledgement of the "divine light" (enigmatic nature) in each individual, and of their successful completion of the ritual. In incorporation, the teacher contextualises the experience from which the students are emerging (by presenting a reading or asking students to focus on a sensation or even through silence). The ritual is completed, and students leave to return to their quotidian lives, although possibly changed. It may take some time for experiences had in a successful ritual to be integrated by the student, but the experience is a personal one and may not be comparable to others' experiences. In rituals, actions become instruments for meaning making and allow for innovation through creative exploration. Without this context, yoga may simply, but successfully, function as a system of fitness, health, and well-being, but students will not be challenged to focus on the meaning of their experiences.

A more obvious opportunity for transformation is found in the progression of a teacher training. It is here that trainers more often recognise the importance of ritual and create meaningful events, which mark stages and changes of status for their trainees. This is because the training has a set duration for completion and clear goals (unlike ongoing studio classes, which lack a consistent clientele). Once accepted for teacher training, a trainee enters the stage of separation, even though this may not be overtly marked. This may be accompanied by a feeling of camaraderie with those who are about to embark on the training process together. Transition begins when the training commences and may be accompanied by the bestowing of ritual objects (training manual, special props, sacred texts, and journals). Throughout the training, aspirants are put through a number of trials (smaller rituals – teaching their first sequence, accomplishing a new skill, or completing a written assignment) that test their dedication and instil the necessary knowledge and skills they will require as teachers. This stage is both protracted (compared to separation and incorporation) and liminal. It may be accompanied by periods of heightened emotion and demands for self-assessment and awareness that are atypical of their everyday lives. There are also physical demands and demands on their time that may be particularly challenging and require that they "ignore" their relationships outside of the training setting. At the conclusion of the transition period, the aspirant is tested when they teach sample classes and through tests of knowledge in the form of oral or written examinations. These trials carry of a high degree of liminality and are potentially rife with emotional strain. The higher the stakes and the possibility of failure, the more potential for transformation the ritual possesses – thus increasing the value of the ritual process. If successful, trainees move onto the final stage, incorporation, which trainers often mark with the most obvious and elaborate ritual action. There is an awarding of certificates printed on special paper, the wearing of ritual clothing adorned with a garland of flowers, and celebratory incantations through which each individual's accomplishments are affirmed. These actions bring about *communitas* – a sense of belonging (Turner 1969) that for some time may connect this group. A well operated ritual will serve as both a Rite of Passage and a Rite of Intensification.

An effective teacher does not manage the student's unique ritual experience but instead facilitates the ritual process. The lasting force of any ritual depends on the authenticity of ritual action. A teacher or trainer creates rituals that are believable and genuinely meaningful to them. It is also important that they consider students' impressionability and whether or not they can convey the appropriate significance of the transformational process through terms that resonate with the student. Affecting or appropriating trappings or pretentions that surpass the magnitude of the transformation is disingenuous and may lead to disillusionment once the heightened emotions of the moment have faded.

THE FUNCTIONS OF RITUAL

Ritual Enactment as Method

In modern settings, the importance of group practice – the *sangha* (community) – may seem in stark contrast to that of the reclusive aesthetic. In order to understand the potential importance of this shift, the function of ritual action in creating communitas will be explored along with the more modern concepts of "flow" – absorbed states of focus and performance (see Csikszentmihalyi 2008 and Schechner 1985) – and "social drama" – where accepted truths are tested within special contexts (Staal 1996). Through these theoretical models and teaching practices, this section will examine yogic practice in light of ritual and performance theory and the relevance this may have in teaching modern yoga. This will illustrate how, if understood as a ritual, a yoga class may become an even more effective site for deep exploration and learning, rather than mimicry.

Yoga, in the anthropological discourse, is understood as a ritual of transformation and sacrifice; ritual that has undergone syncretic changes brought about through the interconnected forces of globalisation and orientalism. (See Mallinson and Singleton 2017; Singleton 2010; Strauss 2005; Jain 2014; et al.). Its roots are firmly planted in the practices of the East; ritual practice demanding sacrifice (austerities) and strivings for transformation have commonly been part of indigenous worship in the religions of the Indian subcontinent. Although yoga is a philosophical enterprise, it is at its core essentially pragmatic – a technology for enlightenment – it is a goal-oriented endeavour.

Yoga as Initiation

Traditionally, yoga is characterised by its "initiatory structure" (Eliade 1969, 5). The student is accepted for tutelage and guidance of a master (*guru*) as in many traditional Eastern disciplines, but yoga takes this initiatory character further in its departure from societal norms – "the yogin begins by forsaking the profane world, (family, society) and, guided by his guru, applies himself to passing successively beyond the behavior patterns of and values proper to the human condition" (Eliade 1969, 5). These rituals "pursue the creation of a 'new body,' a 'mystical body' ... which will allow the yogin to enter the transcendent mode of being ..." (Eliade 1969, 6). This is a mystical rebirth where the yogin experiences an indescribable state of divine being. This strong symbolism of rebirth is also found in the early *Brahmanic* tradition where, by right of birth, some were seen as "evolved" beings, "twice born".

Surprisingly, in its Western forms, yoga as it is practiced in a studio setting, commonly retains this initiatory character. New initiates strive to learn a sacred language (Sanskrit), which identifies them and reaffirms their membership in this select group. Ritual objects are utilised: the harmonium, iconography, singing bowls, gongs, incense, props, and in particular, the mat, which must be kept clean and is reserved for ritual practice. A special etiquette is learned; students regard the studio as a "sacred space", one in which the power of "energies" or "supernatural" forces might be engaged, all to experience "reality" through altered consciousness and to potentially achieve some sort of transformation. An alternate set of rules is invoked in the studio space; there are no shoes, people may touch each other, emotions may be expressed, and people chant together in a mysterious language. These alternate rules may serve to "unsettle" the student and allow them to question the efficacy of the rules in the mundane world outside the studio. The transformational value of this discomfort should not be underestimated.

Ritual provides an opportunity to reframe somatic practice into something meaningful – transformation, in the ritual context, results from the desire for meaning. In addition, ritual creates a liminal (in-between) state, in which a practitioner can be both the actor and observer – doing and watching oneself doing – experiencing and observing that experience simultaneously (see Schechner 1985 and Zarelli 2004). Liminal states promote the experience of heightened and refined sensation and the awareness of these sensations. For example, one may distinguish the intensity of pleasure from that of pain and thereby clarify the two as distinct – intensity will be understood as pain when it is without sufficient reward. Without a way to make meaning, there is no transformation, only suffering. Such ecstatic events are central to the somatic method and are meant to reveal the nature of reality. An example of the reframing of the meaning of intense pain is found in the experience of childbirth. In Western culture, women are now led to believe that pain is best controlled in childbirth. In contrast, if one is predisposed to natural childbirth, they will reassign meaning to pain. The intensity of the experience not only becomes the ecstatic means through which the transformation to motherhood occurs, but also is viewed as a necessary aspect of the success in the ritual transformation. In her article, "Giving Birth, the Endocrinology of Ecstasy," Dr Sarah Buckley asserts that the endocrine system actually responds to the painful birthing process by producing a cocktail of hormones that chemically help induce the blissful state (Buckley 2006). Without the pain, the experience risks becoming simply a medical procedure devoid of the deeper meaning. Likewise, by practising long-held postures, a yogi learns to distinguish between "good" and "bad" intense sensations. This discrimination enables them to explore sensorial intensity in a way that avoids injury, advances knowledge, and reframes "suffering", by giving it meaning.

Yoga as Sacrifice

One only need look to the pages of yoga magazines, sitcoms, digital media, or marketing imagery to see that yoga is now part of popular culture. Even in this modern guise, yoga may retain an initiatory structure; albeit an initiation entrenched in a markedly different culture with different symbols. Popular culture strips away the complexities of form and function as well as the subtleties of meaning, so that it may appeal to a mass audience. It is also, however, a record of a cultural moment, a truly contemporary take on the state of the art. Traditional symbols, reframed and moulded by modern Western sensibility, still exist within a continuum of rules and meanings drawn from Indian culture, which refer to the basic practice of sacrifice central to all ritual transformation. This sacrificial premise, *puja*, can still be seen in modern group yoga practice, where sacrifice is found in the action of performing postures. It is the burning of caloric value, not just an intellectual process; its force lies in its public execution, not simply its conception. Sacrifice implies a permanent alteration, whereas thought alone may be ineffectual or retractable. Traditionally, for instance, the *Bhagavad Gita* describes sacrificial fires and ritualistic practices like *puja*; the preferred sacrifice is symbolised in an internal fire – *tapas* (ritual heat) – to which the literal sacrifices of fire are only alluding (Schweig 2010, 72). To achieve this sacrificial "burning", one applies the proper "skilful" action.

Cross cultural examples of the public nature of sacrificial rituals abound. In her ethnography of Tamil rituals, Isabelle Nabokov contends that "sacrifice is always a public endeavor" (Nabokov 2000, 151); while Christopher Fuller documents both public animal (*bali*) and vegetarian (*puja*) sacrifice found all over the Indian subcontinent as communications with the supernatural world, serving to bring deity and worshippers closer together (Fuller 2004); and Luc de Heusch terms this public striving for union the "conjunctive power" of ritual (2007, 213). Likewise, anthropologists would contend that the shift to a public group practice (e.g., modern classes), further elaborates the ritual and performative nature of yoga where, in such public shared contexts, symbolic meaning is highlighted and elaborated.

Sacrifice Recycles Energetic Potential

In yoga traditions, sacrifice entails the use of heat in practice; the fire is stoked internally at a space below the navel. This fire (*agni*) burns impurities (*ama*) and transforms them into energetic potential. Sacrifice is believed to generate heat (*tapas*) in the body of the practitioner. This heat successfully arises through action, harnessing the qualities of deities, imagination, emotions, powers needed to obtain certain goals, and unleashes a creative force. Since sacrifice implies a permanent surrender of something of value, it destroys but also gives birth to new combinations and new states of being. The sacrificial energy is therefore regenerated, not relinquished. In this way, sacrifice makes room for innovation and growth, and provides the power that fuels transformation.

The process of sacrifice may be undirected or directed. For example, if you apply heat to water, it boils and is transformed into steam. Similarly, if you act, you become the thing that the act predicates – that is the transformation. In modern yoga classes, students are often asked to direct sacrificial practice. Phrases like "dedicate your practice to something important to you" are commonly heard as an entry into the practice ritual. Theoretically, the way the student directs their sacrifice will inspire them to meet culturally specific expectations for transformation, or they may actually effect change. The questions that this poses for teachers are many. How much does intention matter, and should sacrifice instead be "unattached" (Schweig 2010, 63–66) and progress without the expectation of results? To act sacrificially, according to one message of the *Bhagavad Gita*, is by definition a divine act directed at the necessity (*dharma/bhava*) of the action itself; the illusion (*maya*), or misdirection, is to think that one's own actions have impact outside of this reality. As Eliade states of somatic practice and its esoteric meaning: "Through all of his concrete action-gait, bodily posture, respiration, etc. the ascetic must concretely rediscover the 'truths'…he turns all his movements and actions into pretexts for meditation" (Eliade 1958, 167–168).

Eliade suggests that, in ritual movement, one is utterly absorbed; actions are merged with awareness. In modern terms, they are "in the moment". Mihaly Csikszentmihalyi describes this highly focused state of directed function as *flow*. In flow, the most challenging tasks are executed with a minimal expenditure of mental energy. The brain is in a "cool" state. When people are engaged in activities that effortlessly capture and hold their attention, their brain "quiets down" in the sense that there is a lessening of mental arousal.[15] The key to flow is that it occurs only within the reach of one's peak ability, where skills are well-rehearsed, and one does not have to think. Once tasks are mastered, little mental effort is needed to perform them, and then creativity and innovation are possible (Csikszentmihalyi 2008, 111–113). Well-practiced moves take less effort than ones just being learned. It interrupts flow to reflect too much on what is happening – the very thought, "Hey, I am doing really well" can break the feeling of flow. Attention, instead, is so focused that people are aware only of the narrow range of perception related to the immediate task, losing track of time and space. There are several ways to enter flow. One method is to deliberately focus total attention on a task; a highly concentrated state like that achieved through meditation is essential to flow. Entry into flow also occurs when people find something they excel at, and engage in it at a higher level, slightly taxing the limits of their ability. Csikszentmihalyi says, "People appear to concentrate best when the demands on them are greater than usual, and they are able to give more than usual. If there is too little demand on them, people are bored. If there is too much demand on them, they get anxious. Flow occurs in the delicate zone between boredom and anxiety" (Goleman 1986, 1). The implications for yoga as a transformational practice suggest that, if a state of flow (*dharana/dhyana*) is to be achieved, the student will have to be challenged. The experience must be demanding, but within the capacity of the student so that they do not become distracted by frustration.

THE STUDIO IS A STAGE

The studio may be imagined as a stage, where the doorway acts much like entrance into the theatre. "Sacred" objects – mats, altars, candles, bowls, incense, and even blocks and straps – function much like sets and props. Teachers and students take on roles appropriate to the norms of the studio and the yoga community. These are special roles, indicative of their membership in a distinctive group that, to some extent, diverges from larger social norms. Within the studio, actions both challenge and, at the same time, reaffirm cultural norms and beliefs. In this light, the studio serves as a unique venue for what Victor Turner termed the "social drama" (Turner 1980). It is a place where public rituals are played out daily and community is created and reaffirmed. While participating in a ritual, one can be overtaken by their own actions. Deep feelings sometimes emerge that are not quite understood. These emotions may be due to the fact that rituals work; there is no need to understand the symbols or the script to feel them. "It is characteristic of a ritual performance ... that it is self-contained and self-absorbed. The performers are totally immersed in the proper execution of their complex tasks ... even when their purpose is unknown" (Staal 1979, 3). Transformations that result from this emotional experience may be short lived or more lasting. The doing of the actions draws one deeply into them without asking that these actions be comprehended (at the moment of doing).

While successfully performing a ritual, one is in flow; merged entirely within the action. Flow is not unique to ritual, but the repetition and deep familiarity of a ritual, combined with full sensory engagement, help one surrender the "I-self" and to merge with the "Us-self" (Schechner 1985, Chapter 2). Rituals give one permission to *give in*. This same sense, first of self, then of communitas (self, bonded with others), then of the totality (to things even greater) is the goal of ritual in general, and yoga in particular.

Notes

1   Layne Redmond. AZQuotes.com, Wind and Fly LTD, 2021. www.azquotes.com/author/61199-Layne_Redmond, accessed 3 August, 2021.

2   As an illustration, if one's theory is that movement originates in the pelvic region, then a method for testing this would require that instruction for movement be directed from the pelvic region. A technique may be that the action of twisting originates from the hips (rather than some area of the spine or even the shoulders). This can be applied to any postural instruction that involves twisting.

3   Layne Redmond. AZQuotes.com, Wind and Fly LTD, 2021. www.azquotes.com/author/61199-Layne_Redmond, accessed 3 August, 2021.

4   Though originally coined in 1909 (first edition) by van Gennep as "incorporation", others have since termed the final stage of ritual progression as "reincorporation" and "reaggregation" to highlight the fact that change wrought through ritual action returns one to a group with a new status. Also, one may be incorporated with a new status into the smaller group where the ritual occurs without being incorporated into society writ large in a new status.

5   Schechner Fall 2008/Winter 2009 – commenting on Eibl-Eibesfeldt 1979.

6   These practices are also in violation of Eastern traditions, as feet may be considered "unclean". One kisses the feet of the *guru* in order to express overt submission before the *guru's* sacred nature, for even their feet are "clean" in the ritual sense.

7   "In the same way that gold is melted in a pot to remove its impurities, by the virtue of the dirt rising to the surface as the gold boils, and the dirt then being removed, yoga boils the blood and brings all our toxins to the surface, which are removed through sweat" (Jois, 2010).

8   Ayurveda, translated as the "science of life", is the traditional practice of humoral medicine originating on the Indian subcontinent. As one of the *darshans* and yoga's sister science, it shares many underlying principles. Health, for example, is based on a balance of three energies (*doshas*), and illness is the result of imbalance. Ayurvedic doctors employ a number of treatments including dietary, lifestyle and exercise prescriptions to restore balance and, therefore, health. Like yoga, Ayurveda is a practice.

9 According to Ashtanga Yoga (Jois) tradition (Ashtanga Yoga Research Institute 2020), both full and new moon days are observed as yoga holidays – it is reasoned as "natural". Human beings are about 70% water, so they are affected by the phases of the moon. The full moon energy corresponds to the end of inhalation when the force of *prana* is greatest; an expansive, upward moving force that makes one feel energetic and emotional, but not well grounded. Ashtangis look to the Upanishads, which state that the main *prana* lives in the head. During the full moon, people tend to be more headstrong. The new moon energy corresponds to the end of exhalation when the force of *apana* is greatest. *Apana* is a contracting, downward moving force that makes one feel calm and grounded, but dense and disinclined towards physical exertion. It is claimed that practicing Ashtanga Yoga over time makes one more attuned to natural cycles. Observing moon days is one way to recognise and honour the rhythms of nature so one can live in greater harmony with it.

10 According to the teachings of Iyengar Yoga, being on the right can help distribute the blood better through the body with the aid of gravity. One activates the left side of the brain when one moves the limbs of the right side, accessing the thinking mind. From the perspective of Indian culture, the right side is traditionally the favourite starting point, as the right side is considered the more auspicious side in India. It is the right foot that's used to step into a newly constructed building. Items are given and received with the right hand. Even the word *hatha* (ha meaning sun, a right-sided energy, and tha meaning moon, left-sided) places the right polarity before the left.

11 Commonly, students are instructed to roll over onto their right side into foetal position, and then use their arms to help them gently rise to sitting.

12 Various authors describe the meaning of touch and the concomitant rules for touching. See Birdwhistell 1970; Hall 1973 and 1990; and Morris 1997.

13 The stage of transition is not "real" in the sense that one does not live their life in a liminal state. Simply imitating the posture of a yogi in clothing, mannerisms, or speech does not create transformation (as the *Hatha Yoga Pradipika* also states 1.68) (Sinh 1997).

14 Mircea Eliade (1969) gives a description of the distinction between enstacy and ecstasy. Enstacy was coined by Eliade to mean an intensely experienced state of changelessness motivated from within the individual. He contrasted this with ecstasy that was motivated by external stimuli.

15 Marcello Spinella, p.c. 17 April, 2020.

Appendix 2: Reflection and Experimentation

Rituals are commonly employed in everyday acts, although they are often overlooked. They do, however, have a significant impact on the way that we experience reality and manage the mundane challenges of living. For example, we might want to make and drink coffee in the morning as much for its boost as for the ease with which this routine begins our day. There is a security and a familiarity in rituals, and the breaking of routines can disrupt our focus and the normal rhythms of our day. Though breaking routine can lead to novel experience, creating heightened awareness, our rituals allow us to pursue more important tasks at any particular moment. Getting ready for bed helps focus us for the important task of sleeping; chanting *Om* in unison at the beginning of class helps us synchronise our breath with others and prepares us for the important task of practice.

2.1 THE RITUAL SEQUENCE

Write down your personal practice rituals and the rituals you employ in teaching. How do you divide up a class and mark each stage of the practice experience for your students? Are there mini rituals or other techniques or devices you use to highlight certain moments? Analyse the ritual elements in your personal (solo) and group practice. Compare and contrast the experiences as transformative events.

2.2 ROUTINE AND RITUAL

Practising technique is not the same as doing yoga – rather, it is like a musician "warming up" by playing scales before a concert. But, in yoga, the ritual of warming up the body runs the danger of becoming the goal itself. What is your warming up ritual? (When and why do you start it? How does it end? Is there a moment(s) of greater importance?) Is doing a yoga warm up "yoga" and, if so, is it more "yogic" than doing anything else? What is the purpose of this ritualised behaviour, and how do you re-evaluate its potential for deep experience in your teaching and practice? Does yoga have anything to do with sequences or practices, or is it something else altogether – a mindset, an intensity, a devotion?

2.3 RITUAL PROGRESSION IN CLASSES AND TRAININGS

Rituals have three stages of progression: separation, transition, and incorporation. Ritual transformation can be observed and fostered in classes, courses, and training. In teacher training, status change is clear; you begin as a student and end as a teacher (in between you are a trainee).

Rituals need to be culturally appropriate to be genuinely meaningful and transformational. What rituals have you either participated in or facilitated that were memorable in this way? Dissect them to understand the elements of ritual and how they were successfully employed. Consider components of the environment, time of day, props, participants, etc.

2.4 MEANING MAKING: INTENSITY

Sensations are given meaning through experience. We can have different meanings for the same sensation (e.g., pain) in different contexts. How do you understand the "pain" felt in exertion – as in a class with long holds? Understanding this, when is intensity desired? Beneficial? Pleasurable? How many Sun Salutes before the intensity kicks in? Where does your mind go? What problems need to be resolved? What makes intensity easier (e.g., music, the company of others?) and is this beneficial? Pain is easy to experience, but what are other intense sensations that might be explored through practice and how do you effectively experience these?

2.5 SYNCHRONISATION AND RITUAL

Ritual behaviour is stylised, repetitive, and purposeful. Klaus Nevrin (2008, 128) suggests that group practice, when synchronised, is "easier" as it relieves the "burden of individuality". The synchronisation of breath and movement is one way to create ritual action in Sun Salutations. What do you do to synchronise movement and breath in a group class, and how does this facilitate meaning making? How do you expand your and your students' awareness to others in the room? Does one outlier necessarily disrupt a ritual experience? Does this synchronisation make practice easier, and, if so, why?

2.6 YOGA AS SACRIFICE

Sacrifice is an essential aspect of yogic transformation. What sacrifices are made in the service of "tapas" (creating ritual heat) – veganism, time, relationships, your body? What is your austerity, and does it give you delight? What about your practice enables you to consider what is "essential" and what can be stripped away (sacrificed)? How is sacrifice essential to progress in yoga? How will you teach this to your students?

References

Ashtanga Yoga Research Institute website. Accessed 2 August, 2020. www.ayri.org/method.html.

Birdwhistell, Ray. *Kinesics and context: essays on body motion communication.* Philadelphia: University of Pennsylvania Press, 1970.

Buckley, Sarah. *Giving birth: the endocrinology of ecstasy*, 2006. Accessed 10 October, 2020. www.kindredmedia.org/2006/11/giving-birth-the-endocrinology-of-ecstacy/.

Csikszentmihalyi, Mihaly. *Flow: the psychology of optimal experience.* New Yok: Harper Perennial Modern Classics, 2008.

de Heusch, Luc. *Why marry her: society and symbolic structures.* Cambridge: Cambridge University Press, 2007.

Driver, Tom F. *Liberating rites: understanding the transformative power of ritual.* Charleston: BookSurge Publishing, 2006.

Eibl-Eibesfeldt, I. "Ritual and ritualization from a biological perspective." In *Human Ethology,* edited by M. von Cranach, K. Foppa, W. Lepenies, and D. Ploog, 3–55. Cambridge: Cambridge University Press, 1979.

Eliade, Mircea. *Yoga: immortality and freedom,* translated by Willard R. Trask. New York: Pantheon Books, 1958.

Eliade, Mircea. *Yoga: immortality and freedom.* Translated by Willard R. Trask. Princeton: Princeton University Press, 1969.

Fuller, C.J. *The camphor flame: popular Hinduism and society in India.* Revised and Expanded Edition. Princeton: Princeton University Press, 2004.

Geertz, Clifford. "Deep play: notes on the Balinese cockfight." *Daedalus* vol. 134, no. 4 (Fall 2005): 56–86.

Goleman, Daniel. "Concentration is likened to euphoric states of mind." *New York Times.* (4 March, 1986): Section C, Page 1.

Hall, Edward T. *The hidden dimension.* New York: Anchor, 1990.

Hall, Edward T. *The silent language.* New York: Anchor, 1973.

Huizinga, Johan. *Homo ludens: a study of the play element in culture.* New York: Angelico Press, 2016.

Jain, Andrea. *Selling yoga: from counterculture to pop culture.* Oxford: Oxford University Press, 2014.

Jois, K. Pattabhi. "Introduction." *Yogamālā.* New York: North Point Press, 2010.

Mallinson, James and Mark Singleton. *Roots of yoga.* London: Penguin Classics, 2017.

Morris, Desmond. *Intimate behaviour: a zoologist's classic study of human intimacy.* Tokyo: Kodansha Globe, Reprint Edition, 1997.

Nabokov, Isabelle. *Religion against the Self: an ethnography of Tamil rituals.* Oxford: Oxford University Press, 2000.

Nevrin, Klaus. "Empowerment and using the body in modern postural yoga." In *Yoga in the modern world,* edited by Mark Singleton and Jean Byrne. London: Routledge, 2008.

Redmond, Layne. *When drummers were women.* Three Rivers Press, 1997.

Schechner, Richard. *Between theater and anthropology.* Philadelphia: University of Pennsylvania Press, 1985.

Schechner, Richard. "A ritual seminar transcribed." *Interval(le)s* II.2-IIL.1 (Fall 2008/ Winter 2009): 93–116.

Schweig, Graham M. *Bhagavad Gita: the beloved lord's secret love song.* New York: HarperOne, 2010.

Singleton, Mark. *Yoga body: the origins of modern posture practice.* Oxford: Oxford University Press, 2010.

Sinh, Pancham, trans. *Hatha Yoga Pradipika.* New Delhi: Munshiram Manoharlal Publishers Pvt Ltd, 5th Edition, 1997.

Staal, Frits. "The meaninglessness of ritual." *Numen,* vol. 26, issue 1 (January, 1979): 3. https://doi.org/10.1163/156852779X00244.

Staal, Frits. *Rituals and mantras: rules without meaning.* New Delhi: Motilal Banarsidass, 1996.

Strauss, Sarah. *Positioning yoga: balancing acts across cultures.* Oxford: Berg, 2005.

Turner, Victor. *The forest of symbols.* New York: Cornell University Press, 1967.

Turner, Victor. "Liminality and communitas." In *The ritual process: structure and anti-structure,* 359–374. Chicago: Aldine Publishing, 1969.

Turner, Victor. "Social dramas and stories about them." *Critical Inquiry* vol. 7 no.1 (1980): 141–168.

van Gennep, Arnold. *Rites of passage,* translated by Monika Vizedom and Gabrielle L. Caffee. Chicago: University of Chicago Press, 1960.

Zarelli, Phillip. "Toward a phenomenological model of the actor's embodied modes of experience." *Theater Journal,* vol. 56 (2004): 653–666.

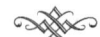

CHAPTER THREE

TEACHING SOMATIC PRACTICES OF YOGA
THEORY, METHOD, TECHNIQUE, AND FORM

TOOLS FOR TEACHING

This chapter will consider concepts for general teaching and the more specific demands of teaching a somatic practice, by providing the foundational knowledge needed to teach any style of physical yoga. First, the principal components of body dynamics and the relationship between mind and body will be discussed in a brief overview of embodiment theory and some fundamentals of kinesiology and principles of movement. Next, the notion of *levels* will be considered through the theory of *pedagogical approximation*[1]. A detailed discussion of the four basic components of teaching – *theory, method, technique,* and *form* – will follow, bearing in mind the importance of their hierarchical relationship. Finally, the chapter will conclude with applications of theoretical perspectives on teaching and learning.

EMBODIMENT AND SOMATIC PRACTICE

Many in the somatic disciplines have written brilliantly about the science of embodiment. At its core, embodiment rejects the Cartesian dualism of mind/body and presupposes that the mind and body are part of the

DOI: 10.4324/9781003181910-4

same interactive entity; mind and body impact one another. As Merleau-Ponty writes, "the body is us. We are not simply our minds." In fact, experiences in our bodies create who we "are" (Merleau-Ponty 2002). Embodiment is a way of thinking about bodily experience – it includes pleasures, pain, suffering, vulnerabilities, capabilities, constraints, and sensorial and sensual engagements with the world, as they arise within specific times and places. It is both the experience of *corporeality*, of living in and through the body, as well as *phenomenology*, the philosophical study of conscious experience from an individual's subjective perspective (Wilkerson 2015, 67). In short, we become who we are through our experiences in our bodies. Embodiment may be described then as the degree one feels that they fully inhabit their body. Disembodiment, by contrast, would describe a degree of bodily disengagement, separation, or dysphoria. When we increasingly engage with our bodies, we are able to have more heightened levels of experience in which we see ourselves as full human beings (Zarelli 2004, 661).

The Phenomenology of Spirituality

Sociologist Emile Durkheim noted that the rise of *spirituality* was a function of modernity.[2] Spirituality, he contended, was "the triumph of individuality over religion" (religion being formalised in social institutions) and arises in cultures that value individualism. Spirituality has therefore been understood as a unique, individual enterprise, one in which experiences lie outside of the influences and institutions of society. More recent studies suggest, on the contrary, that spirituality is very much a part of cultural institutions and that these institutions provide ways for spirituality to be expressed and validated. Courtney Bender, in her ethnographic study of metaphysical practitioners in Cambridge, Massachusetts notes that "what we think of as spiritual is actively produced within medical, religious, and arts institutions, among others. It is not unorganised or disorganised, but rather, organised in different ways, within and adjacent to a variety of religious and secular institutional fields that inflect and shape various spiritual practices" (Bender 2010, 23). This is not to diminish the value or authenticity of spiritual experience (or the existence of divine energy or supernatural forces), but simply to say that engagement with them is culturally mediated, as is the meaning made from these experiences. Before Pythagoras theorised the Earth was round, direct experience demonstrated unequivocally that it was, instead, flat; and it still does. The reality of the Earth has not changed, but the experience has been reimagined by the change in knowledge that altered *worldview*. Examples of the imaginative and interpretive nature of direct experiences abound cross-culturally.[3]

We see or commune with God or nature or supernatural realms according to our expectations gained through the process of enculturation and ongoing socialisation. Envisioning chakras, colours, bright light from the third eye, or the beauty of a sunset; experiencing bliss/love, free-flowing energy, or connection to something larger than ourselves – these are all real experiences, but they are not unadulterated. They are conditioned by our worldview and the ways we have learned to make meaning. Yoga practitioners, for example, may experience seven *chakras*, acupuncture practitioners envision energy either flowing or obstructed along the meridians, and reiki healers connect to the free-flowing energy fields to balance the energies of their clients. But various yogic texts have proposed four to nine *chakra* systems, and practitioners in all these metaphysical vocations have conflated the differences in their experiences to be "all about the same energy", despite the fact that they understand energy in distinct and disparate ways.[4]

Yoga is based on experience; it is foundational and of utmost value. In particular, what should we make of spiritual experiences; those that entail direct connection to divine entities or the ethereal? A definition of *spiritual* is fraught with ambiguity, but, here, it will be understood as any individual experience concerned with the essence of life, spirit, or soul. Spiritual phenomena are immaterial and, therefore, defy scientific explanation or reification. Spiritual experiences are *real* and very valuable in that they may provide comfort, motivation, perseverance, and the ability to withstand adversity. They are important vehicles for the imagination, providing different perspectives, fostering creativity, and conceiving alternate possibilities. They can provide comfort and a sense of belonging by encouraging connectedness and promoting feelings of joy, bliss, or ecstasy. But, to mistake these experiences as outside the influence of preconception, or to validate students' experience as an objective truth in the teaching of yoga, is irresponsible. Doing so promotes *groupthink*,[5] limiting students' ability to evolve or imagine other perspectives or realities. Groupthink can also become a habit of mind, where students cease to question beliefs held within their practice community, let alone question the teacher. Such a state of mind erases the possibility for healthy scepticism and critical discussion.

Embodied States: Kinesthesia, Rehabituation, and Flow

Psychologist Maxine Sheets-Johnstone (1999) proposes that the way we move has an impact on how we feel about our bodies and our environment, because movement and attention to movement can produce a heightened sense of awareness and less stressed sense of identity – a less rigid sense of self (Smith 2002). In other words, being embodied allows us to imagine the possibilities for personal growth, learning, and evolution. If attentive movement can create a greater sense of fluidity, an ease in moving about in the world and more easily adapting to challenges and changes, what impact might a lack of movement or a lack of mindful movement have on one's sense of self? From this psychological perspective, lack of movement is debilitating. Depression, for example, is exemplified by a number of somatic sensations, not the least of which are bodily pain and an overall sense of weightiness. As Bartenieff explains, "…depression is often experienced in the body as a passive giving in to weight. The slightest movement can diminish this. What is important is the indication of participation, rather than passivity" (Bartenieff 1980, 157–158). The recognition of two states enlisting both the mind and the body, stillness and passivity, is noteworthy. So powerful is the smallest movement (even passively performed) that it will cause a chemical reaction in the brain and decrease the symptoms of depression. When movement is performed deliberately (a patient spends time on a treadmill for instance), the impact is significantly greater. This is part of a larger phenomenon called *rehabituation*; when the way one experiences the world is changed simply by learning new ways of using and making sense of one's body (Sheets-Johnston 2010).

Examples of the power of rehabituation as a tool for teaching are myriad in yoga. Generally, the attainment of a posture, like a headstand, which once seemed impossible, can provide ongoing motivation for learning and dramatically open a student's mind to larger possibilities for their practice. Internal dialogues, like "my stomach is too big" or "my arms are too weak", are replaced by self-talk that reflects confidence in their abilities, the process of learning, and the feasibility of change. Moments where these accomplishments happen can be intensely felt, especially when they are unexpected. Rehabituation requires self-assessment and, although an accomplishment may be first felt with a rush of adrenaline or excitement, change requires that the experience be internalised. Students may need time to process their accomplishments and a teacher may lose the opportunity to capitalise on the power of somatic experience by applauding or otherwise drawing undue attention to these accomplishments, especially in a public context (like a class or workshop where others applaud). Teachers can, instead, quietly acknowledge the gravity of a student's accomplishment and provide ongoing encouragement so that rehabituation may take place through the integration of experience.

The phenomenon of rehabituation can be understood from the perspective of neuroscience, as it describes actions of the brain – how consciousness is altered – in various undertakings that produce the feelings engendered during and subsequent to physical accomplishments. In prosaic tasks, sensory information that is nonessential is inhibited to ensure the required focus and attention necessary for successful completion. If the task is sufficiently easy, however, sensory information that is peripheral to the task is permitted into awareness (Austin 2010, 373–407).[6] This could also be couched in terms of hemispheric difference. According to Iain McGilchrist, the left hemisphere of the brain sees the world in terms of "utility." Therefore, its perspective is that one's *will* is about *control* such as we find in the execution of physical tasks. If our disposition toward the world is altered to a right hemispheric perspective – if it becomes one of *care* rather than control – "[i]ts will relates to a desire or *longing* towards something, something that lies beyond itself, towards the Other" (McGilchrist 2009, 171). There is an undeniable abstract beauty in such theoretical constructs (as there is with the Tantric imagery of *koshas* and *nadis*), but the practitioner seeks intense, focused experience and not an explanation of conscious processes. How to facilitate this state of conscious awareness is one concern of the teacher.

In a somatic practice like yoga, the teacher aims to utilise techniques that facilitate some level of altered consciousness through embodiment. These states of consciousness range from the fully alert kind of analysis engaged in working out where to place limbs while observing the demonstration of a posture, to an inner imagining of "subtle body" landmarks, through possibly hypnogogic states in Corpse Pose. *Vinyasa* adds to this the particular consciousness of "flow" discussed in the previous chapter (and elaborated below). In Chapter 1, two extreme standpoints for practising physical yoga were considered – one that negates the body/mind and one that affirms it, but virtually all practice occurs on a spectrum between these. Just as the degree of somatic involvement is relative, so too are the kinds of consciousness found in the experience of yoga. Altered states of consciousness are likely to occur for the serious practitioner and these directly correlate with the body's experience, but students need to understand them in their own terms. The practice of physical yoga deliberately uses the body to influence the state of consciousness to create such unusual experiences. Therefore, the teacher facilitates changes in consciousness through body positioning, movement, and context, rather than attempting to directly manipulate students' thoughts or interpret their mental states. As Nevrin (2008, 123) notes, immersing oneself in movement can (through diligent training) take the form of "sustained dynamic flow" that is normally not experienced in everyday forms of body performance. It may be "experienced as an elongated or ongoing present, it is a world in which there are no befores or hereafters, no sooner-or-laters, no definitively expected endings or places of arrival" (Sheets-Johnstone 1999, 151).

If one experiences a particular sense of well-being in Corpse Pose, is this because the experience is only possible in this position? Or is it possible to also experience it in other parts of practice under more challenging circumstances? When the movement in *vinyasa* is continuous, evenly metered and follows the breath in such a way as to create a state of equanimity, it approaches that state sought in Corpse Pose. Evenness of breath coupled with evenness of movement (both sequential or holding) results in evenness of mind and is therefore achievable throughout practice.

Embodied techniques are found in all somatic practices and high levels of embodiment are consistent with high levels of holistic bodily awareness known as *kinesthesia* (Sheets-Johnstone 1999, 152). In a kinesthetic state, common to great athletes, the individual is aware of their body as a single entity in space, and therefore can move it more gracefully, efficiently, and effectively. This is why they are perceived as "hardly trying" or "making it look effortless". In fact, those with high levels of kinesthesia expend less energy, often feeling increased stamina after exertion rather than feeling depleted.

Closely connected to whole body awareness is the state which Mihaly Csikszentmihalyi defined as *flow* (Csikszentmihalyi 1990).[7] Flow is a mental state of operation in which a person performing an activity is fully immersed in a feeling of energised focus, full involvement, and enjoyment in the process of the activity. Flow is complete absorption in what one does, with intensely focused motivation, and a single-minded immersion; it represents the ultimate experience in harnessing the emotions in the service of performing and learning. When one is in flow, emotions are not just contained and channelled, but positive, energised, and aligned with the task at hand. The hallmark of flow is a feeling of spontaneous joy, even rapture, while performing a task, although flow is also described as a deep focus on nothing but the activity – not even oneself or one's emotions.

The harnessing of emotions to achieve "peak experiences" can be best understood through a clearer definition of *emotions*. In this context, emotions will be defined as the physical expression of a psychological state; as *feelings*, or intensely felt states of mind. For example, one can direct emotional energy – joy, anger, excitement – toward the goals of practice using this same energy as motivation. The intensity of emotion will corollate with its impact. Many in the yoga community prioritise some emotions over others; joy and happiness are good emotions; anger, on the other hand, is a bad emotion and should be controlled through "nonreactivity". It is the position here, however, that emotional content of any kind can serve to heighten experience and that emotions are useful when they are an appropriate "felt sense".[8]

Hyperfocus

Hyperfocus has many of the same characteristics as flow (highly focused concentration, intensity of experience), however, it is not always described in such glowing terms. For example, some cases of spending "too much" time playing video games, or of getting side-tracked and pleasurably absorbed by one aspect of an assignment or task to the detriment of the assignment in general. In some cases, hyperfocus can "grab" a person, perhaps causing them to appear unfocused or to start several projects but complete few. This poses a number of interesting questions for yoga teachers. Among them: Can a practice suffer from hyperfocus to the detriment of the prospect for flow? What percentage of practice should be focused on technique and can technique get in the way of the peak experiences that are sought for students? Does single-minded striving for perfection lead to paralysis? Keeping in mind the goal of peak experience, teachers decide how to utilise the process of hyperfocus so that it serves as an effective tool. Flow requires a high level of challenge that, at the same time, avoids frustration. Understanding "where the student is" is essential to providing the proper level of difficulty to facilitate the intense experiences that allow for learning, advancement, and peak performance.

Neuroscience and Altered States

In her doctoral thesis, studying the meditative experiences of Zen Buddhist practitioners, Aska Sakuta looks to neuroscience to understand altered states achieved in embodied practices. Sakuta notes the central importance of the "meditative, attention training processes, embedded in the act of movement" in various somatic disciplines, from dance to theatre, and within other performance styles:

> ...within this process of meditative moving, the mover experiences an altered state of consciousness, which can be expressed as the state of 'no mind' – a sense [of] complete emptiness of the mind. It is thought that the strong concentration on the felt experience of moving facilitates a state of deeply embodied consciousness by stripping the mind of distracting thoughts. The mind, thereby 'emptied' of higher level cognition, allows for movement execution at the most intuitive level.
>
> (Sakuta 2017, 1)

This intuitive execution of movement is akin to the state of *flow*, a state of deeply embodied consciousness acquired through training in techniques (specific to each discipline). Once mastered, these allow the practitioner to achieve peak performance through altered sensory states involving "[self-initiation], focused concentration, internal sensing, elimination of distraction, and releasing objective judgement of performance outcomes" (Sakuta 2017, 2). A deeply embodied state of consciousness is defined by Sakuta and others as a set of feelings or sensations arising during that state, including "an effortlessly sustained attention, the loss of self-consciousness, and a sense of automatically arising movements." This state is achieved through practice in a series of stages beginning with effortful concentration (cognition), advancing into "optimal movement economy" (embodiment), culminating in "complete automation" (phenomenology), where the body seems to move on its own; the experience may be described both as effortless and spiritually charged (Sellers-Young, cited in Sakuta 2017, 3). The relevance of this perspective to somatic yoga practice is obvious, as is the neurological functioning of the human brain that makes these experiences possible (see Austin 2010).

The notion of efficiency of movement is worth exploring more deeply as a way of understanding embodied yoga practice since it helps us to understand the conundrum posed above about technique and the potential pitfalls of hyperfocus. What Sakuta and others suggest is that learning technique is a necessary stage in the process of mastery that allows for optimal movement and only after such knowledge is mastered – integrated into one's body/mind – can movement occur naturally and a meditative state be achieved. This is embodied as ease of movement and may be observed aesthetically as "grace." It is this grace that in *vinyasa* practice may be likened to seamlessly moving with both attention to and in response to one's breath.

Grace

Can we experience spiritual grace through graceful movement? A definition of grace is action performed in a way that is energetically appropriate to the circumstances – too much effort and it appears strained; too little and it is ineffectual. Although "graceful movement" might be described as "effortless" by a casual observer, they are misled. Practitioners know that robust action is needed to accomplish difficult tasks gracefully. In *vinyasa*, grace is not just doing challenging movements, but also how adept one is at gauging the interaction between the personal and external circumstances. Awareness of these conditions deftly guides the amount of effort expended on breath, physicality, and mental focus. (Even a simple act of greeting by shaking hands is difficult to get just right – it involves "reading" the circumstances. One doesn't pump the hand of someone's auntie the same way you would a tough guy in a bar.) The teacher is tasked with how to teach grace and equanimity through challenging movement. They encourage the student to keep a cool head and to act with a poise unique to that student. It is more than just efficient – it is apposite. Similarly, describing it as "no mind" or "unconscious competence" or "empty" (Sweeny 2009 in Sakuta 2017, 1) might also be misleading if grace of spirit is equated with "flow" state. In flow, one knows who they are and can perform to the best of their capability; on some level they identify what is essential and eliminate the superfluous. The same could be said of spiritual grace. Someone who has grace would have no need to express it through the trappings of dress, mannerisms, or forms of speech – they are what they essentially are – a unique amalgam of everything in their past, what is happening to them now, and that which could potentially occur. The individual could try to enact this "essentiality" in a restrictive manner through an ongoing process of refinement towards inaction of the mind/body; or, alternatively, in a performative manner, through creatively participating with the complexity of that which appears to be Other. This is not an either/ or situation – it is a question of deeming which method is most fitting and engaging with that in an energetically appropriate fashion. Grace, whether it be physical or spiritual, requires that a person knows "who they are" and acts in a fashion that applies no more or less than that.

Mastery of technique is something that is first taught in the controlled environment of a studio where sequences of movement or postures are repeatedly visited. These simple movements are practical and arise from proper body dynamics as they are practiced in everyday life. However, as yoga movements increase in physical difficulty or complexity, their use outside the studio in work-a-day reality lessens. It would be difficult to make a case for the practical application of inversions. The teacher's job is to clarify how mastery of unusual movement leads to creative and spontaneous problem solving beyond the studio. One way to approach this is to make the material sufficiently challenging so that things go "wrong" for the practitioner – requiring that they adapt without losing their "grace". If someone loses balance in a posture or a sequence, they are afforded an opportunity to actually practise yoga – to keep breathing smoothly; to plausibly and economically re-engage with what they were attempting without the loss of equanimity.

Surrender and Control

The term *hatha yoga* denotes forceful action, so what is one to make of the emphasis placed on *surrender*? As stated above, it requires great effort to achieve a state of intense experience in somatic practice – entailing control of the breath, control of the body, and control of the mind. Surrender may be applied, therefore, to all that is not essential; that which will distract the practitioner from the unification that leads to grace. This begs the next question: How does one know what is not essential? In *hatha yoga*, when instruction encourages the cultivation of focus (on breath, mind, and body), the practice of surrender will be discovered through experimentation and attunement (constant observation of one's body/mind). Control through this method makes surrender possible; it is a realistic proposition attained through the process of discrimination. Yoga practitioners surrender what is counter to their purpose, but exactly what is surrendered will be dependent on the method of practice and the theory (underlying principles) on which it is based.[9]

Time

There is a contention in yoga literature and practice that "we are not the body", and "neither are we the mind"; yet we are something incarnate in the body. The "something" that we are is characterised as being exactly the same as the essence of the universe. This singular essence that unites the Totality or the Absolute is variously referred to as *Brahman* or, perhaps more poetically, as consciousness or *purusha*. This essence is said to be something that is "unchanging", "eternal", and "indestructible". Time is irrelevant because it is always the same – not differentiated in any way – the passage of time does not alter it, so it is irrelevant to consider before or after with regard to it.

How does a yogi's body and mind – both firmly entrenched in the temporal – come to terms with experiencing this consciousness that is beyond time? Traditional *asana* yoga techniques have sought to immobilise the mind and body (as well as the breath) and, when the energy (or *prana*) of these is made latent, then the yogi is able to experience what remains. *Vinyasa* posits that the state of consciousness found in "flow" gives an insight into what this timeless state is and likens this to the experience of beauty where there is a Self-awareness.

The Intimacy of Breath

The practice of yoga adds an important component to embodiment theory – attention to and control of breath. Breath is the communicative link between mind and body. Breath awareness serves to examine oneself by revealing the connection between mind and body. How does breath change our sense of embodiment? Attention to breath changes the experience one has in one's body (phenomenology)[10] through the use of techniques like shifting focus, assuming imaginative or emotional states, and varying intensity. In addition, the manipulation of breath with directed attention or through techniques of *pranayama*, intensifies the effects on the body and the mind reciprocally, resulting in a fuller sense of embodiment. For example, if one lies with their eyes closed and imagines only breathing through their right nostril, they will automatically give greater attention to the right side of their body and "feel it" differently. Breath is an intimate expression of being; an indicator of internal and external status at any moment. One of the most intimate experiences one can have with themselves is found by listening to and attending to one's own breathing. This is intuitively understood by even the most novice of students, for upon entering a studio for the first time, their major anxieties are generally about requests to go barefoot and breathing audibly in class. It could be argued that these are "odd" behaviours in public, and that is certainly correct, but other important symbolic associations are attached to these behaviours for Westerners. Bare feet are usually only acceptable in private settings (no shirt, no shoes, no service) much like any sort of "nudity" (and also for reasons of hygiene). Even more so, when one can hear another person breathing, it is often in the context of intimacy. This certainly helps to explain why new students are reluctant to produce audible breathing. Revealing the sound of one's breath is just that – revealing. The intimacy that is experienced is awkward when compared to that which occurs when one is alone or in a private context. Sometimes these contextual boundaries are confused and students will make other noises, which they might only make in private spaces – moaning, for example.[11] Observation of breath is an invaluable tool through which the teacher is able to survey the student's internal state during practice.

Teaching Breathing in Somatic Practice

Yoga teachers are often heard saying things like, "Focus on your breathing", "It's all about your breath", and "Let your breath lead your practice"; but what do they mean? It is hard to know, especially since breath specific to somatic practice is rarely taught outside of designated *pranayama*[12] instruction. *Ujjaiyi* breath is most often associated with physical practice. Jois' Ashtanga Vinyasa offers some specifics to indicate how breath and movement are linked. But, even here, little direct instruction in breathing is given; nor the manner in which breath is associated with the *bandhas* or energetic locks.[13] There are other techniques for performing *ujjaiyi* breath, which facilitate changing states of consciousness and also follow modern anatomical principles.[14] Whatever techniques are used, they should be clearly understood, practiced, and presented by the teacher in the service of the goals for practice.

What happens in the brief time that exists in the change between inhale and exhale? One can certainly admire the beauty of poetic replies to this that suggest this brief suspension gives insight into the "space between our thoughts" – a suggestion that between the overt search for embodiment that *vinyasa* cultivates through its evenly metered breath, there may also be another "suspended reality" that is not body or mind. It invites intriguing interpretations. Is there a way to combine the ethos of *asana* yoga with its negation of the body and mind with *vinyasa*'s full-on affirmation? Can one (or does one without knowing it) fluctuate between these two premises and technically control the entry and exit from each? It is an area that could stimulate fruitful experimentation – deliberately lengthening the pause between breaths to induce an altered state of consciousness. How might such fluctuations affect feelings of well-being? How would they impact on the skill levels exhibited? How does it impact aesthetically? There is a multitude of questions concerning the breath that require ongoing experimentation and can greatly enhance the experience of discovery in practice.

BODY BASICS: KINESIOLOGY AND THE KINETIC CHAIN

There are many ways of describing body dynamics that may be applied to understanding the physiology of movement in yoga. These concepts are useful as tools for analysing students' form and movement. Here, a few kinesiological models are presented that may enhance a teacher's ability to "see" both a student's capabilities and what they might do to safely and efficiently discover their potential. The concept of *kramas*,[15] which we refer to as *levels*, suggests that all things can be broken down into their significant parts or levels of enactment. Though Krishnamacharya understood these levels as components of set sequences of increasing difficulty, they might also be defined as deconstructions of postures, movements, or complex concepts that preserve their important effects and underlying principles. The concept of levels and teaching based on an evaluation of each student and what they are "ready to hear" is a way of recognising a student's somatic intelligence. What are the skills required to perform this *asana* (posture, movement, etc.)? Can I break down this *asana* into its component parts? Can I discover levels that encourage both understanding and learning for my students? Can I apply these levels to create appropriate and effective variations? Levels may also be applied to proven teaching methods like *repetition* and *scaffolding* (repeating a skill in different ways and in different contexts). Likewise, concepts can be presented directly and simply, creating an environment that is challenging but not frustrating for students. One figures out the levels of a posture or movement in their own practice through precise attention to movement, and the deconstruction of this movement when performed in concert with breath. For example, in a seated forward bend, a teacher may instruct those with tight backs or hamstrings to keep their legs active while bending their knees, to facilitate an accessible hinge at the hips on the exhalation (Figure 3.1). From here, students can inhale to lengthen the torso and exhale to hinge and progressively move toward straightening their legs. For those that are flexible, teachers may have students raise their heels on blocks or reach around a block in front of their feet in the same active manner. By bending the knees, the teacher can decrease the difficulty of the posture, reducing the amount of abdominal strength and the hip and back flexibility required to straighten the legs. This knowledge may be used to create many variations of forward bends to encourage the experience sought in any forward-bending posture.

In applying levels to teaching, one is most effective working within the principles of *pedagogical approximation,* which is defined here as a system for determining how much information and what kind of information you use to instruct students (from beginner to advanced understanding).[16] For example, real beginners might be offered more global or general information that suits the building of foundational knowledge. As students advance, the teacher may determine that they are ready for increasingly complex, detailed, or subtle information. Giving a student excessively detailed or overly complex information may serve to frustrate or lead to misunderstanding (which inhibits the desired state of flow). Pedagogical approximation requires constant evaluation and *attunement,* where teachers evaluate students' understanding throughout the teaching and learning process. A teacher must deliver information that is accessible and relevant, even if it is initially a simplification or exaggeration used to illustrate a point less subtly. The teacher sets the parameters for each student's level of investigation – weighing and evaluating their current capabilities and potential for understanding – including sensitivity and need. Each correction,

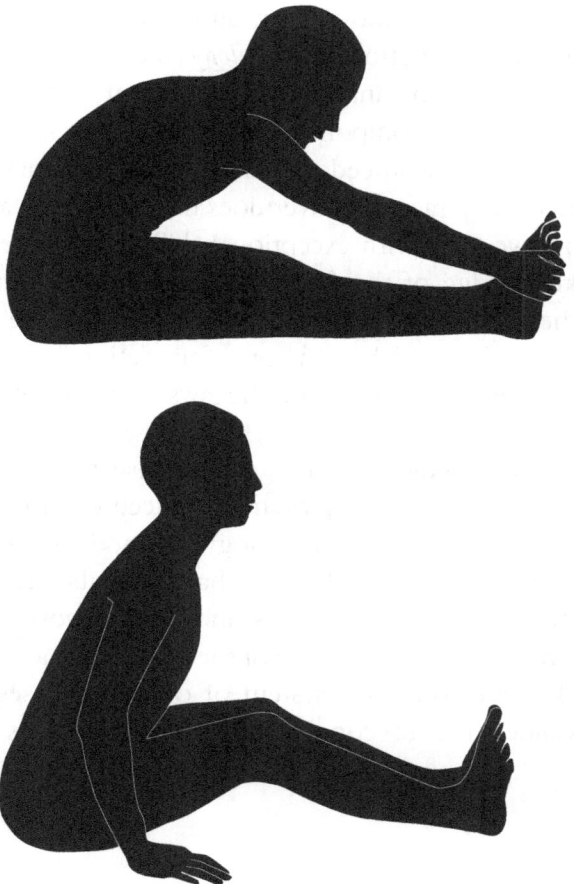

Figure 3.1 Seated Forward Bend modification

and its presentation, is a form of experimentation on the teacher's part. Teachers may find the employment of metaphors useful to describe a more subtle point in concrete, more easily accessible terms (e.g., an inhale may be described as "opening your ribcage like an umbrella"). Properly delivered information encourages students to "keep at it" even when the postures or movements are not yet within their capabilities. Good teaching reveals the skills that are necessary to achieve these postures and movements, and provides a clear route to progress.

Efficiency of movement is an important component in the mastery of any somatic discipline and may be defined as: moving while expending only the necessary amount of energy, the effort of which is distributed throughout the entirety of the body. Enlisting the entirety of one's being in the service of an action is a function of focused concentration, understanding breath and movement, and a holistic understanding of the body's structure in motion. *Kinesiology* (the study of how the body moves) is interested in the anatomy of movement, rather than discrete anatomical landmarks or components like bones, muscles, and joints. As embodied beings, humans need not know structural anatomy to learn how to move, just as a race car driver does not have to be a mechanic to know how to drive a car with exceptional skill.[17] What they both need, however, is knowledge of the functioning of the instrument they are moving. In the case of the yoga teacher, this knowledge is *functional anatomy*. This section will look at two foundational aspects of functional anatomy: the kinetic chain and the laws of spinal rotation and side bending.

Kinesiologic knowledge encourages the coalescence of the body required as a foundation for exploration of deeply embodied states of consciousness. One concept in kinesiology is a model of body dynamics called the *kinetic chain*.[18] The kinetic chain describes the interrelated groups of body parts, connecting joints, and muscles working together to perform movements, and the portion of the spine to which they connect. It views the human body as a system of overlapping segments (e.g., hand-arm-shoulder-ribcage) connected by a series of joints (Figure 3.2).

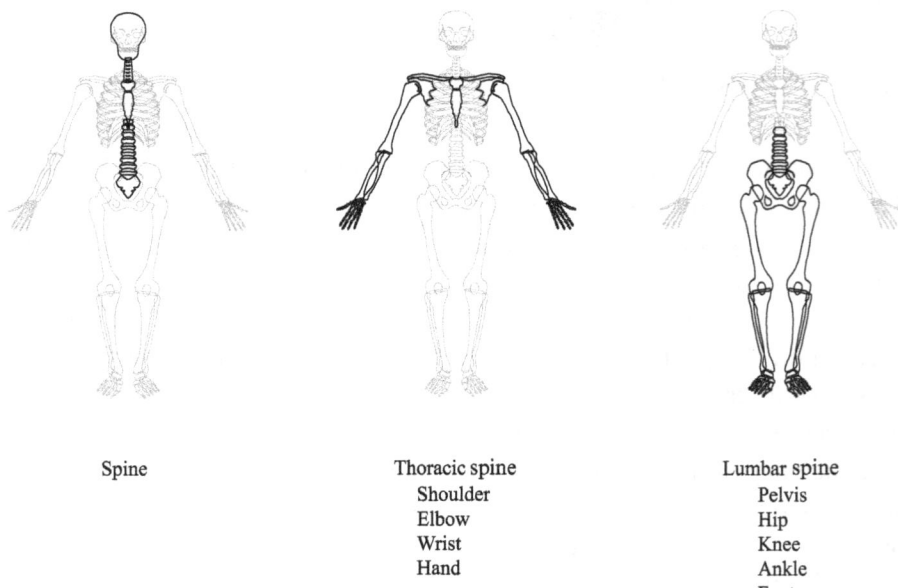

Spine	Thoracic spine	Lumbar spine
	Shoulder	Pelvis
	Elbow	Hip
	Wrist	Knee
	Hand	Ankle
		Foot

Figure 3.2 Principal kinetic chains

Movements occurring within each segment are expressed in either *open-chain* or *closed-chain* patterns – dependent on whether the distal end (furthest from the spine) of the chain is fixed or free to move without restriction. Open-chain movements are those where the distal end of an extremity moves freely in space – such as when one raises their hands over their head or if one's feet are suspended above them in a headstand. A closed-chain movement refers to a position where the most distal part of a given extremity is fixed to the ground or another solid object, which results in the body moving about the fixed joint. Once movement is initiated, the repositioning of the joints and surrounding musculature – moving through the chain – are modified due to this fixed position. For example, when the feet are planted on the ground during Lightning Pose (*utkatasana*),[19] the rest of the leg chain (ankles-knees-pelvis-spine) will move towards the fixed end of the extremity – the feet – as the body lowers into the squatting position (Figure 3.3).

Closed-chain movements promote joint stabilisation and have the potential to recruit more muscles and their associated joints, encouraging somatic integration. Open-chain movements involve more shearing forces at the involved joint compared to closed-chain movements and tend to recruit the musculature associated with only a single working joint, resulting in less integration. Students unknowingly may modify their postures in an effort to conform to "making the right shape" – unknowingly, because this modification may be inappropriate for their

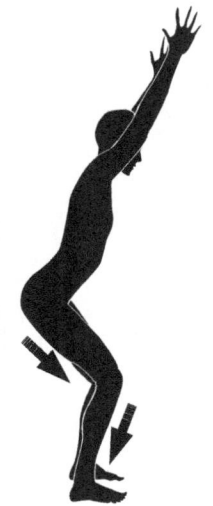

Figure 3.3 Lightning Pose and closed chain

functional anatomy. For example, in Warrior I, a student may turn out their front foot, increasing the external rotation of the same hip, so that they may go more "deeply" into the posture. This deepening seems desirable to the student because they mistakenly see wider legs with the thigh parallel to the ground as "better". In fact, this is only a geometric imposition on an organic form; the student's true Warrior I is achieved in a stance that is in accord with their anatomical structure and capacity to fix the position of the front foot while squaring the hips (Figure 3.4).

Another example is when students turn their front foot inwards when practising Twisted Side Angle (Warrior) (Figure 3.5). This increases the internal rotation of the hip on the same side and provides a wider frame for balance. This may allow a student to enter a deeper twist because, in disengaging the hips that normally act as the centre of gravity, the spine

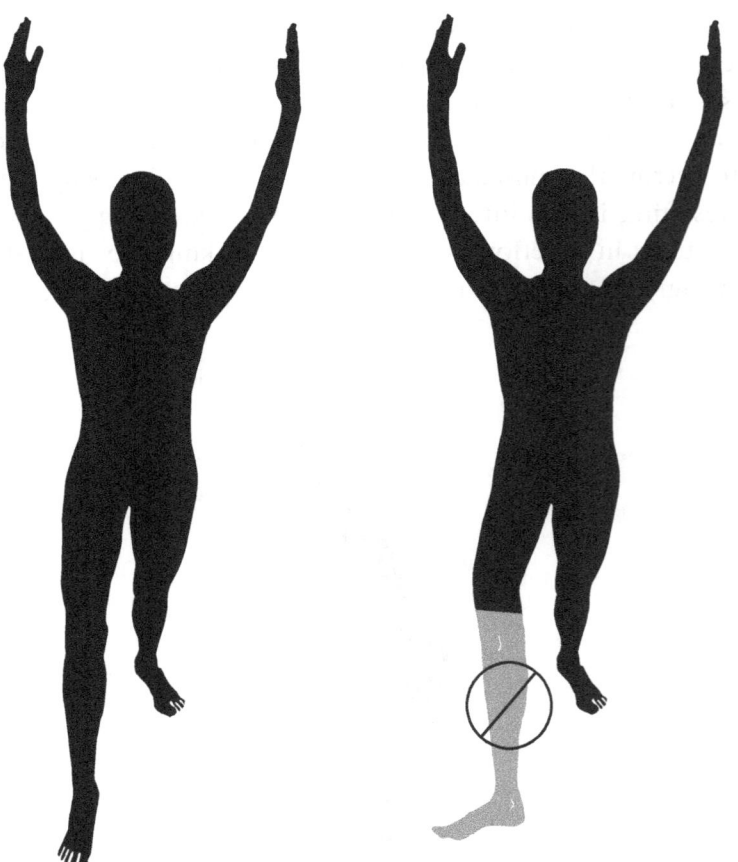

Figure 3.4 Warrior I Pose

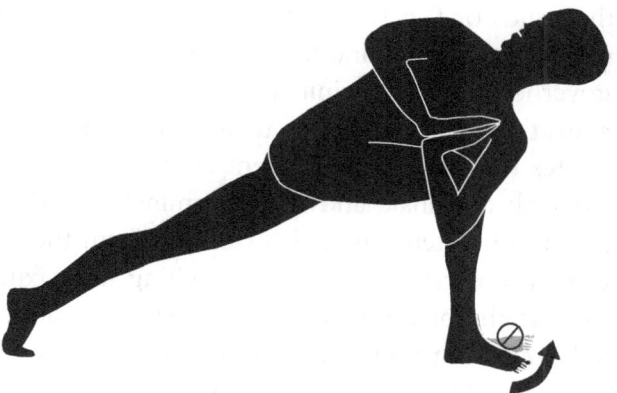

Figure 3.5 Twisted Side Angle Pose

curves, weight is shifted to the front foot, and the structural integrity of the knee and groin are compromised. This accommodation occurs (and is sometimes taught) to enable a student to make a "shape" (get the elbow on the outside of the thigh or the hand on the floor), all at the expense of sound body dynamics. Instead, students should be encouraged to keep their hips engaged and only twist as far as this engagement can be maintained. This perspective on teaching arises from the theory that postures create effects and are not unassailably idealised shapes – that yoga is practiced to achieve grace in the mind/body.

In yoga practice (and in teaching yoga), we attempt to engage the entirety of the body. From the perspective of the kinetic chain model, all actions would then approximate closed-chain movements – even when the more distal portion is not secured on a surface of some kind. This involves utilising techniques that mimic a closed chain by enlisting the muscles and joints of a chain in a way that creates resistance; as if the distal portion is positioned on a stable surface.[20] For example, when one balances in Warrior III, they reach through the elevated leg as if they are pressing it against a wall. This engages the lower chain as if it is one unit, allowing it to work in unison. It is this integration (along with continued hip engagement and the resistance to gravity achieved by pushing the floor away with the standing leg) that enables the student to balance.

This introduces an important refinement of the kinetic chain model when it is applied to yoga practice. Because yoga seeks to integrate the body/mind into a unified whole, imagining the body as two chains linked together through segments of the spine may be too fragmented. What is it that unifies the upper and lower chains and the spine? It is not where one places the hands or feet (as the kinetic chain model may suggest), but what *happens* to the hands and feet because of the action of the hips; and this is governed by what is initiated by the mind and the breath. When one transitions from standing to a high arch in a Sun Salute, the mind initiates the forward movement at the hips. This movement is coordinated with an inhale and the abdominals lengthen while the thighs are drawn into extension. This extension from the centre of the body radiates to both distal extremities, reaching its maximal point at the same time that the breath reaches its fullest expression. The whole body is unified in creating a high arch through this process. The entirety of the body is engaged to some degree in any performed action, within or outside of yoga practice; it does not work segmentally in natural movements. This is the essence of embodiment; in yoga, the level of awareness of the unified body/mind gives us insight into the nature of self.

It follows, then, that the kinetic chain also needs to include what is between each link: the muscles, fascia, ligaments, tendons, and other anatomical structures. Instability in a joint will create instability in the joints closest to them and along the chain (proximally and distally). When the teacher creates variations for the purpose of either instruction or execution, it is important to recognise that mobility in a joint will affect mobility in the next joint in the kinetic chain. Flexion in the elbow supports flexion and rotation in the shoulder; flexion in the knee likewise increases flexion and rotation in the hips. Therefore, a teacher can make a posture or movements more accessible for students with tight hips or shoulders by creating variations with the knees or elbows bent or passing through bent positions towards straightening (bent limbs still must be instructed so that the whole of the chain remains engaged). This knowledge allows a student to experience the connections within their bodies, facilitating higher levels of embodiment.

Stability and Flexibility

Certain joints in the chain are meant to be stable and others mobile for alignment and movement. Teachers should instruct with the functional movement and support for each joint in mind, so that students gain an understanding of increased stability and avoid injury.[21] Yoga requires a balance between mobility and stability. However, stability and strength are prerequisites for *developing* flexibility. One cannot lengthen a muscle efficiently or increase long-term flexibility without a stable base from which to "stretch" one's muscles. Stability is created by engaging and coalescing the whole of the body, on each breath.[22] Stability may be taught through active muscular resistance, oppositional movement (pushing and pulling), and activating the whole body in postures and movements, among other techniques. The muscular actions needed to accomplish *ujjayi* breath will result in bodily integration if consistently practiced. The intention of somatic practice is to foster optimal functioning so that the body may act as an instrument for physical and spiritual exploration. When flexibility is valourised at the expense of strength, it jeopardises this optimisation.

The Law of Rotation and Side Bending in the Spine

The spine rotates and bends in predictable ways depending on whether the segment is lordotic (concave) or kyphotic (convex). The *law of rotation and side bending* designates that in the cervical (neck) and lumbar (lower back) sections of the spine, which are lordotic, side bending rotates the head of the vertebrae in the same direction as it bends (spinae rotate in the opposite direction).[23] In the thoracic (upper back), which is kyphotic, side bending rotates the head of the vertebrae in the opposite direction of the bend (spinae turn in the same direction). This knowledge allows teachers to understand how to deepen a posture without creating compression in the spine (Figure 3.6). For example, if one is teaching a standing side bend, the shoulders will turn in the opposite direction of the bend and the pelvis will turn toward the bend to find the maximum side extension; likewise, in postures such as Triangle and Side Angle. When a teacher disregards these kinesiological rules, they constrain students' ability to explore the physical and experiential depth of a posture and risk injuring them.

ASSISTING, ADJUSTING, AND SEQUENCING

Assisting and Adjusting

Teaching requires that students are guided through practice using both encouragement and critical assessment. If a teacher is to assist or

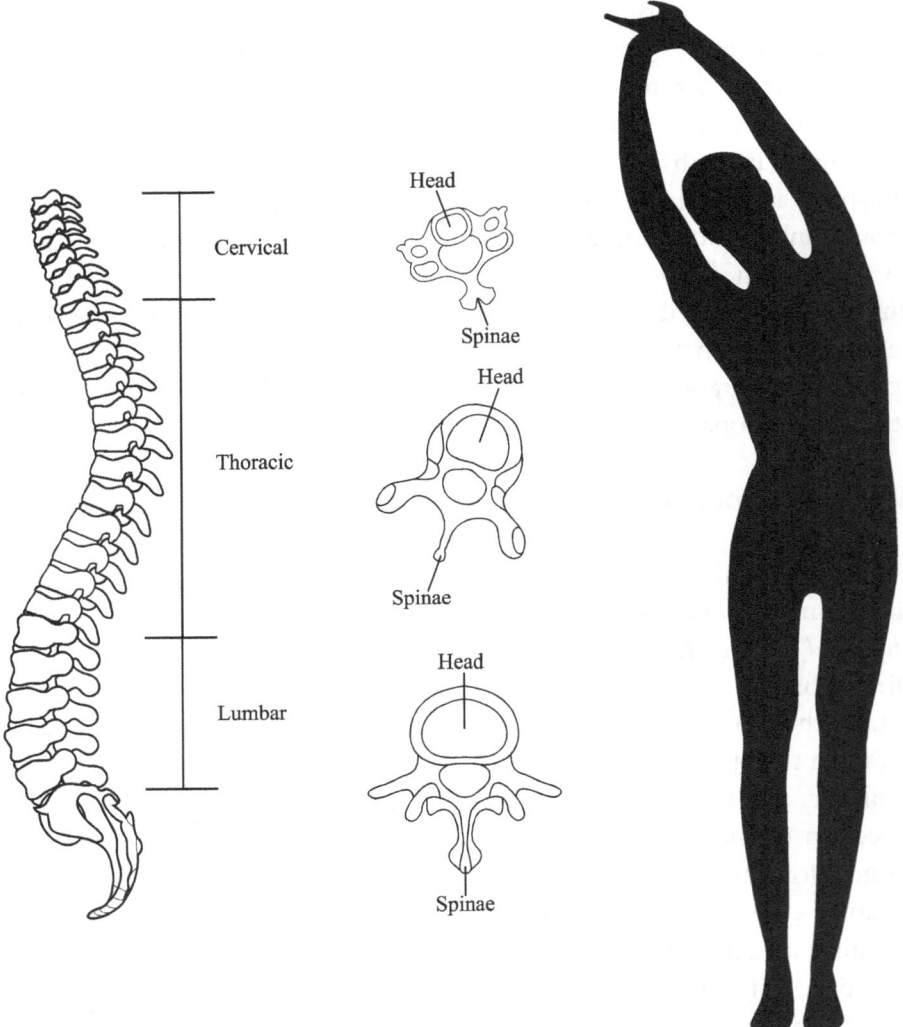

Figure 3.6 Law of Rotation and Side Bending

adjust, they must do so with a strong knowledge of functional anatomy. Without this knowledge, teachers could either physically impose or verbally encourage unnatural shapes or movements on students' natural functional anatomy. *Adjusting* is the most common directive given by teachers; it can be the verbal, demonstrated, or physical correction made to a student's alignment, postural comportment, or movement. Adjustments may also act as encouragement rather than merely corrections of form – supporting students in their continued exploration and improvement. *Assisting* is a more invasive alteration of a student's form, which is meant to achieve a position through the hands-on intervention of the teacher. This includes various instances where a teacher might support (inversions and balances) or deepen postures (twists, connecting binds, or forward bends). Neither assists nor adjustments are meant to encourage dependence on the teacher, but rather to reveal to students what is possible in the exploration of the next level of the posture. Assisting and adjusting are both methods for teaching; not strategies for expressing care or giving attention. Gratuitous use of corrections risks fostering dependency instead of furthering the student's knowledge and increasing their sense of agency in the development of their practice.

Assists and adjustments are often thought of as codified, but utilising standardised corrections belies good teaching for a number of reasons. First, different interventions are needed for different problems that students have in executing either techniques or form. Second, assists and adjustments are employed in the service of teaching; therefore, what and how a correction is made is wholly dependent on what is being taught at that moment. For example, if one is teaching students the importance of engaging the hips in a lunge through the expression of the exhale breath in the legs, adjusting arms that are askew would be a waste of a teaching moment. Instead, adjustments might encourage students to drive the back hip forward and extend through the back leg as it internally rotates and the lower back integrates. This directs students to experience the intended instruction and use their own bodies as sites for experimentation. Third, because each teacher's and student's body is different, each assist or adjustment should be unique, since it must take into account their comparative height, weight, and structure.

A common way to assist a student is through demonstration. The ability to accurately demonstrate a Sun Salute or a posture is an easy way for people to initially learn something novel. The teacher who undertakes to instruct and refine that which they cannot do must have considerable ability and knowledge to explain a movement or make adjustments. Hence, demonstration is a useful tool which requires that a teacher maintain the integrity of their own practice and have a deep understanding of what they teach. Yet, when a teacher is in the midst of demonstrating, they cannot have their focus on what a student is doing, so they are careful to balance demonstration with observation.

Sequencing

In teaching somatic practice, sequencing is not arbitrary, as every *asana* or movement should be practiced in a specific way for a specific reason, at a specific moment; practice without purpose is not yoga. This is true regardless of the system one teaches. A well-structured sequence presents an experiment that the student undertakes to experience a concept proposed by the teacher. This sequence should contain only elements that have contextual relevance and nothing "gratuitous", (e.g., that cool posture learned last week). To be meaningful, sequential elements function to elucidate the concepts or method on which the experiment is based or to prepare students for this experiment in both body and mind. Both fixed sequences, and those uniquely structured by the teacher, have value when they are arranged in a thoughtful, purposeful manner.

Although postures are often viewed as having "standard" effects,[24] the manner in which a posture is expressed, and the sequencing of postures (what precedes and follows it), has much to do with the particulars of this effect. In other words, a posture has no static, consistent set of effects. Manipulating the way in which postures are presented will alter their effect. A headstand may, for example, be "invigorating" or "calming" depending on whether it is practiced with eyes opened or closed; performed through a sequence of variations or held in stillness; sequenced at the beginning or at the end of a longer practice. The degree to which a practitioner is actively working the breath (e.g., *ujjayi*) or manipulating/holding the breath will determine whether forward bends are "cooling" or not. A passive holding practice can be restful or challenging, depending on whether it is practiced in deep unsupported variations (Paul Grilley's Yin Yoga),[25] softly, with the support of props (Sarah Powers' Yin Yoga), or as a restorative sequence (Iyengar). Twists are "balancing" only if they are practiced symmetrically on a symmetrical body. If a practitioner is tighter on one side, practising asymmetrically (holding and deepening on the tighter side) may be balancing, while practising symmetrically may increase imbalance.

The concept of symmetry often goes unexamined. Most practices instruct that postures should be held evenly on both sides and that symmetry is defined through this "balance". Orthodoxies commonly prescribe that postures should be held for five breaths each. With the perspective of critical acceptance, a teacher may instruct a student to re-evaluate the "balance" of symmetrical practice; advising them to create "harmony" in their movements. This might be accomplished by practising in a way that creates symmetry through unequal patterns of holding (spending more time opening a tight hip as opposed to a loose one). Likewise, balancing strength and flexibility may be viewed as symmetrical practice. This highlights the variant concerns of a personal practice and one performed in a group. Moving in unison in group practice provides the opportunity to ease individual burden and facilitate a focus of connection. While this may necessitate global instruction and symmetry, a personal practice is driven by more individual concerns, and is an opportunity for practitioners to explore notions of harmonious movement.

Further complicating the effect of postures is their complexity. Most postures are not easily categorised. Lightning Pose (*utkatasana*) is a standing posture, a forward bend and a backbend, as is Warrior I. The effect of the posture is created through the emphasis of the teaching, rather than a simple essential quality or any "sacred geometry" it may be claimed to possess.[26] Postures may also be understood to have a number of ranked effects: primary, secondary, and tertiary. The degree to which each effect is realised depends on the existing conditions in the practitioner. Those with tight hamstrings will experience almost any forward bend as a hamstring stretch first, despite the fact that this may be the intended secondary effect of the posture. Therefore, if the teacher wants to have elongation of the spine to be the principal function of the posture, they must find a modification that "neutralises" the hamstrings; possibly by bending the knees. Take Downward Dog for instance; if the primary effect desired is length through the spine, the secondary length through the hamstring and the tertiary creating a lightness through the abdomen (*uddiyana*), then the teacher may instruct a student with tight hamstrings to continue to work the legs with knees bent, enabling the torso to lengthen. In short, the teacher selects the sequence of postures and guides students through the manner in which the posture is performed, to achieve the desired effect, in accordance with the "lesson". This manner may be different for individual students even in the same class. To accomplish this requires keen observational skills and entails that the teacher practice the posture in many different permutations, taking note of the effect on their own body in each. The deconstruction of postures into levels amounts to physical experimentation, which leads to a deeper understanding of what one is teaching.

Theory, Method, Technique, and Form

So, where is this purpose found? Rationale for yoga practice is found in one's *theory* and *methods* and enacted through *techniques*. Any *form* one chooses to teach reflects these principles and serves as the grounds for experimentation. In short, a theory of practice determines why one is teaching yoga in a particular way; it includes a clear definition of yoga and the philosophy and goals for practice. The method (*vinyasa, asana,* meditation, *pranayama*, style, orthodoxy) one uses provides the vehicle for testing the validity of the theory on which it is premised as one strives to reach one's goals. Techniques are developed to teach the kind of skills that must be mastered to enact the method in a way that is fully embodied. The form that one teaches should always be consistent with one's theory and method and be performed according to the techniques being mastered. For example, Iyengar Yoga is premised on the *theory* that one can achieve enlightenment through the perfection of alignment on a cellular level; as Iyengar is said to have stated, "alignment equals enlightenment." The Iyengar *method* (Iyengar 1966) emphasises the holding of postures with specific structural alignment to achieve this enlightenment (in addition to many health benefits). Iyengar *techniques* provide detailed points of reference for placement and positioning so that proper alignment may be achieved (the proper positioning of the fingers and toes, the tucking of the tail bone in positioning the pelvis, geometrical relationships between limbs and their relationship in space, etc.). The *form* is a fixed canon of postures and the exploration of these may be made clear and accessible through the use of props (many invented by Iyengar himself for this purpose), which are a component of Iyengar *technique*.

The importance of teaching a practice that is founded on cogent and consistent principles cannot be overstated. When teaching forms (e.g., Warrior II or Tree Pose), if one has a specific alignment, it should be justified through one's theory and method, and enacted successfully through specific techniques. The explanation for teaching alignment should never be tautological. When teaching lateral postures like Warrior II, Triangle, Side Angle, or Half-Moon, if the instruction is "to open your hips to the side wall" (laterally), the justification for this technique to achieve alignment cannot be "because these postures open your hips laterally". Similarly, if one teaches specific foot positioning, there should be a reason for this that is not simply "because that is the alignment" or "that's the way I was always taught" or "because the heels always need to be on the ground". These answers suggest that the teacher adheres blindly to alignment techniques without the knowledge of why they are practiced or sufficient testing of these techniques for validation. What teachers must do instead is employ critical acceptance to anything they have "learned" and establish a theory, method, and set of techniques for their own teaching that are sound and tested through practice.

ADVANCING STUDENTS IN PRACTICE

The teacher is charged with advancing a student by helping to make them more embodied and aware of their internal state based on an assessment of their capabilities and potential. *Capability* is a subjective term that is often misunderstood, as is *advanced practice*. The student's capability is determined by their current state of knowledge, current physical state, current mental state, motivation (aspirations), determination (work ethic), and how regularly they practice. Advanced practice is defined here as practice that develops on increasingly subtle levels; it is not the ability to achieve a posture (shape), it is not inversions, nor is it being the strongest or most flexible. It is the ability to understand the workings of one's mind and body at deeper levels, it is the ability to control and channel one's breath for different purposes, and it is the ability to regulate one's own practice to fit one's needs from moment to moment.

There are generally three types of students: those who think they are less capable than they are, those who think they are more capable than they are, and those who have a realistic assessment of themselves. A teacher's assessment includes recognising the limitations of a student's physical structure and state (injuries, anatomical anomalies), mental state (fear, over-eagerness), as well as their habits (level of discipline, degree of concentration, and their relative distraction with details rather than integration). The teacher also recognises or encourages students to approach their yoga practice as a lifetime development dedicated to the appreciation of the uniqueness of each moment. A practice may mature as the body/mind goes through the ageing process. The teacher acknowledges these changes (both what improves and falls away) as a way of highlighting the importance of this process for their students. *Asanas* and *vinyasa* sequences are not goals in themselves, but tools to affect the body and mind. Practice is about achieving a certain perspective or effect and not postural shape. A*sanas* are human inventions (many very recent) and there is nothing inherent in these shapes that is beneficial; rather, the benefit is in the particular manner of execution.[27]

Testing

Teaching requires testing; teachers give information and test. The test is integral to assessment and at the foundation of advancement. Students learn who they are and their capabilities through a realistic understanding of the outcomes of the testing provided by teachers. Many disciplines require considerable technical mastery because, in pressured situations such as sports competition, the martial arts, or live performance, there are professional expectations. Things that one can do in practice must be replicable. This creates psychological pressures that are anticipatory, such as "What if I fail?" or fear of injury. Rather than concentrating on the actions that need to be done, the mind skitters off into constructs of the future. The focus is meant to be on the here and now. In yoga classes, some students fall apart if they think the teacher is watching them or they fabricate ideas that the other students are "competitive". Advancement comes when focusing on the task/action at hand, not through imaginary catastrophes or competitions with others. It is the teacher's role to redirect the student's attention so that they can prove to themselves their proficiency.

Notes

1 The term *krama* was most famously popularised by Krishnamacharya and later expounded by his student and devotee Swamirama. The term pedagogical approximation refers to the way that teachers choose the amount of information to deliver to students, the method of delivery, and the complexity of concepts, based on an ongoing evaluation of the students they are teaching.
2 See Durkheim (2008), originally published in 1912, for more on the functions of religious practices and the differences between spirituality and religion.
3 See Metcalf (1992) for an overview of the many ways that the spirit world is imagined cross-culturally, or even the nature of reality itself.
4 See Bender (2010) for a detailed discussion of the way that the metaphysical community sees their work as congruent.

5   The term is attributed to George Orwell, *1984* (1949); and popularised by William H Whyte, Jr. "Groupthink", (Whyte 1952). Irving Janis elaborated on Whyte's analysis, "I use the term groupthink as a quick and easy way to refer to the mode of thinking that persons engage in when *concurrence-seeking* becomes so dominant in a cohesive ingroup that it tends to override realistic appraisal of alternative courses of action. Groupthink is a term of the same order as the words in the newspeak vocabulary George Orwell used in his dismaying world of *1984*. In that context, groupthink takes on an invidious connotation. Exactly such a connotation is intended, since the term refers to a deterioration in mental efficiency, reality testing and moral judgments as a result of group pressures" (Janis 2010).

6   James Austin's theory of Egocentric and Allocentric Systems suggests that performing prosaic tasks processes information through a dorsal route to the cortex and inhibits or permits sensory information to get the task done. If the task is sufficiently easy, however, sensory information that is not essential to the task is processed in a ventral pathway, and involves interaction between non-frontal cortical areas, the limbic system, and cerebellum, which makes the neural processing more deeply implicit as less effort is expended on focusing on the direct action of the task. Austin, J.H., "The thalamic gateway: how the meditative training of attention evolves toward selfless transformations of consciousness", in "Effortless Attention" in *A New Perspective in the Cognitive Science of Attention and Action*. Edited by Brian Bruya (A Bradford Book, 2010), 373–407.

7   Colloquial terms for this or similar mental states include: to be *in the moment, present, in the zone, on a roll, wired in, in the groove, on fire, in tune, centred,* or *singularly focused.*

8   According to ancient texts, yoga does not distinguish between good or bad. In fact, the yogic texts suggest that the practitioner should treat each with equanimity. This certainly should apply to emotional responses, since there are times when one should feel appropriately happy, sad, joyful, or angry.

9   In Yin Yoga methods (see Grilley 2012; Zink 2012, Clark and Powers 2012; and others), muscular engagement is discouraged. Therefore, a student is instructed to surrender control of their body (to gravity) and breath control, so that one can maintain "stillness". Their theory holds that this method leads to a meditative state and achieves purported health benefits.

10 *Phenomonology* is the philosophical study of conscious experience from an individual person's subjective perspective. It is meant to serve as a corrective to Cartesian Dualism, which posits a strict dichotomy between body and mind. Feminist scholars see gender as phenomenological, positing that bodily normativity is "masculine and constant" and therefore bodily changes (especially those associated with women – menstruation, menopause, childbirth, aging) are regarded as forms of risk, disturbance, breakdown, and irrationality. Seen through the lens of disability studies, these same bodily changes are "a horizon for self-understanding," and they, along with critical race and post-colonial approaches to embodiment,

argue against Western notions of personhood as "rational and disembodied" (see Wilkerson 2020, 67–68).

11   It is certainly true that some teachers encourage moaning and other expressions of release in class. These behaviours are apt to make some students uncomfortable, as they recognise them to be intimate or private gestures and inappropriate for a public context.

12   *Pranayama* is often taught as a separate practice outside of physical yoga. One exception to this is found in Kundalini Yoga, where breathwork is the practice and movements are made with little precision and without postures in order to wake up *kundalini* energy and clear energetic channels.

13   Pattabhi Jois used the phrase "free breathing with sound" when referring to how we should breathe during practice. The soft sound that is sometimes heard comes from deep within the chest rather than from a restriction in the throat. In practice, he taught that one should aim to keep the inhales and exhales the same length and of even intensity throughout each cycle of breath. Jois described the locks as "squeezing" up the anus (mula) and the lower belly (*uddiyana*) (Jois 2010). No other instruction is given.

14   In *ujjayi* breathing, the physical movement of the inhale breath is initiated with a lengthening of the abdominals (*uddiyana*), which facilitates the opening of the lower ribcage, but which does not interfere with the descent of the diaphragm. This lengthening continues and becomes more extreme as the breath fills so that the upper chest is also expanded. At the same time, the scapula wrap around the side ribs and are drawn down, which promotes the expansion of the back ribs so that the whole ribcage expands uniformly towards its maximum. This abdominal length on the inhale has the tendency to draw the region of the mula forward and preserves the length of the lumbar back. This means, if one is standing, the legs will tend to move into extension so that the muscles of the back of the legs help to draw the lower pelvis down, which also preserves the length of the lower back. The mental image follows a similar kind of expansion – it begins at the *mula* and conceives of energy as radiating outward from that point to the body's extremities at the same rate with which the breath fills. There is an imagistic synchronisation with what the body and breath do. The exhale also uses an *uddiyana* action. The physical movement again begins at the *mula*, but to accommodate the abdominal lengthening, the *mula* now tends to move back in space. The scapulae continue their action of wrapping around the ribs and pulling down, and are a force that aids in closing the ribcage. Mentally, the *uddiyana*'s upward movement is paralleled with the idea that the exhale is a movement of energy from the *mula* outwards towards the body's extremities coordinated with the breath. In both inhale and exhale the jaw is opened, but the lips closed, and the glottis held in a pre-yawn position. Two things should be noted here. First, the *uddiyana* action does not achieve the full expression of *uddiyana* such as it can do when the diaphragm is drawn up on the breath retention that follows an exhale, though it does try to

get close. Second, there is a difference between *uddiyana* and *uddiyana bhanda*. The abdominals are engaged in completely different activities. *Uddiyana bhanda* is not used in *ujjayi* breathing. The abdominals are lengthened on both the inhale and exhale, while in the *uddiyana bhanda*, they are drawn into contraction, which would inhibit the fluid movement of the rib cage. While the merits of *bhanda* for movement of energy in the "subtle body" are strongly held by those inclined towards this structuring of their mental processes, the sustained lengthening of the abdominals in the physical practice of *vinyasa* is done to ensure protection of the lumbar region because it does not allow it to change shape during the extreme movements of the practice.

15 *Krama* is Indonesian for "caste", suggesting the nature of the whole may be understood in terms of its essential parts. Just as castes are immutable components of human existence that support the larger cosmology.

16 This perspective is similar to the teaching methods found in the *Upanishads*, where progressively adept students who are capable of differential understanding are offered different kinds of information by the attuned *guru*. Three categories of students are recognised in "*upanishadic* learning": "ready to listen", "ruminating on teachings", and "synthesising information". Each student will be offered different information based on the subtlety of the questions they pose to their *guru*. These questions are indicative of the level of understanding of each student and the basis for evaluation by the *guru* and the process of attunement.

17 Knowledge of anatomy is a tool that may be useful in teaching, especially if what one is teaching is a therapeutic application of yoga. Understanding movement, however, only requires that one understand functional anatomy, how the many parts of the body support and affect one another as they coordinate in movement.

18 In 1955, when Dr. Arthur Steindler adapted the theory of Franz Reuleaux, a mechanical engineer.

19 Although we avoid using Sanskrit names for postures in this volume, the name is used here for clarity.

20 Attempts to engage the entirety of the limbs and integrate them into the body with breath is accomplished by engaging the distal segment in a posture from the centre of the body. This is usually the hands and feet, but could be the shins (*ustrasana*), the forearms (*pinchamayurasana*), or upper arms (*sarvangasana*). This allows the upper (arm) and lower (leg) chains to move as one, even when the distal portion of the chain is technically "open". Similarly, when a portion of the body is against a stable surface, it must be consciously engaged (pressed away from the centre of the body) to achieve the desired integration.

21 Joints are made to be used for the following purpose: The ankle, hip, and thoracic spine are built for flexibility and a broad range of movement. The knee, lumbar, and cervical spine are built for stability, which must be maintained to avoid injury.

22   The inhalation breath expands the body to make space. The exhalation breath deepens every posture as it integrates the body. This is true with every posture, in any context, when *ujjayi* breath is performed.

23   This is derived from Fryette's Law; a set of three laws pertaining to skeletal anatomy named after Harrison Fryette, D.O. The laws are defined as a set of guiding principles used by practitioners of osteopathic medicine to discriminate between dysfunctions in the axial skeleton.

24   Iyengar yoga states general effects for standing postures (stabilising, energising, and heating) forward extensions (cooling, quieting, and soothing), revolved postures (introverting, leveling, and heating), backward extensions (stimulating, energising, and heating), inversions (calming, regulating, and replenishing), and restorative postures (restful, soothing, and renewing). Though these are overall effects, Iyengar also lists specific effects for each posture.

25   Paul Grilley and Paulie Zink recommend this method and technique.

26   Sacred geometry ascribes symbolic and sacred meanings to certain geometric shapes and certain geometric proportions. It is associated with the belief that a Great and Intelligent Universal Force of Consciousness is the Geometer of the Cosmos (Calter 2008).

27   There is little evidence of the ancient nature of most *asana*, therefore shapes are arbitrary, and creativity and experimentation are encouraged in practice (to achieve certain effects). See "An accounting of the history of yoga" in Mallinson and Singleton 2017; Singleton 2010; Foxen 2020; De Michelis 2005; and Jain 2014; among others.

Appendix 3: Reflection and Experimentation

Teaching the somatic practice of yoga requires an eclectic range of knowledge, including principles of anatomy (structure, movement, and breathing), embodiment (the lived experience within the body), and meaning (spiritual, social, psychological, and aesthetic). Effective methods of delivery and assessment (pedagogy) distinguish yoga teachers from practitioners. These include corrections that offer honest critiques, encouragement, and pathways to success. The exercises below are meant to hone these skills and provide a way to assess and improve the effectiveness of your yoga teaching.

3.1 GETTING INTO THE FLOW (THE PUNK VERSION)

Johnny (Lydon) Rotten of the Sex Pistols once sang, "anger is an energy." Is it necessary to leave anger and your other worries outside the door when you come to practice yoga? "Negative" emotions are often demonised in the yoga community, but a practitioner or teacher can use these emotions (like actors and punk singers do) to perform at a higher level of commitment or intensity. Although emotions can be a distraction to one's effort, especially if they are expressed habitually, critical observation of emotional response creates a mindful observation of expressed emotions in practice.

If expressing emotion brings dissipation (whereas repression perpetuates it) and, in flow, emotions are "channelled" in the concentrated service of one's efforts (Csikszentmihalyi 1990): How would you set parameters as a teacher to best channel students' emotional energy in practice? Should a teacher be required to hide their emotions and be a neutral instrument? Why or why not?

3.2 REPETITION AND VARIATION

Principles are well taught when they are repeated in a variety of contexts. Ideally, each context is used to either reinforce a concept or to introduce new aspects sequentially. For example, you might choose to teach internal rotation of the arm in the shoulder joint when drawing the arms behind the torso. This may be applied to weight-bearing postures like Shoulderstand, as a way to release the neck in Camel or Bridge Poses, or as the foundational concept in binds (in postures like a bound Triangle, or reverse prayer in Warrior postures, etc.). In each case, the same principle is applied in different ways to reveal why internal rotation provides stability when the arms are moved behind the torso. In well-structured scaffolding technique, teachers, through progressive repetition and varying contexts, enable students to make their own sense of related concepts.

Devise a scaffolded sequence (as is illustrated above) in which knowledge of a principle is reinforced as its complexity is revealed.

3.3 EBBS AND FLOWS

Each class/practice has a trajectory. In terms of vigour, classes often peak near the beginning, especially if they start with Sun Salutations, and then slowly wind down. Scaffolding, which keeps circling back to a peak experience or a point of teaching, is a way to progress through a class and perceive that, despite the ebbs and flows of intensity and focus, the experience is continually deepened.

How do you go about scaffolding in your practice and teaching? How does this strategy create and then clarify meaning?

3.4 DECONSTRUCTING AND RECONSTRUCTING PRACTICE

Postures may be broken down into their component parts, a process that we have denoted as "levelling". For example, forearm balance (Scorpion) requires both shoulder flexibility and stability, and the knowledge of techniques for getting into and remaining in balance. Working on each of these elements separately allows students to build skills and experience progress.

Pick a complex or difficult posture and break it down into its important component parts. What does a student need to access the posture (e.g., strength, hip stability, hamstring flexibility, breath control)? How would you teach this posture to students of differing experience, physical capabilities, and bodily structure? How might you incrementally reconstruct these components to move students to achieve fuller expressions of this posture? How would you advance a student that has not yet achieved this posture? How might this be used in teaching "all levels" classes with a diversity of students?

3.5 REHABITUATION

Rehabituation is the process by which we change our sense of self or our abilities as the result of a significant bodily experience. All of us have had experiences – ecstatic to traumatic – which we remember as "life changing events" (e.g., learning to ride a bike, doing your first headstand, giving birth, traumatic injury).

Recall a physical experience that *positively* changed your sense of self. What did this accomplishment entail and how did you achieve it? How might you apply this insight to move students past roadblocks in their practice? Recall a *negative* physical experience; how did you keep this experience from curtailing your progress in yoga?

3.6 TECHNIQUE VERSUS FLOW

Teaching requires a combination of "practice" in techniques and the "performance" of them. In yoga, technique practice is a preparation for achieving the experience of yoga in a flow state (Csikszentmihalyi 1990). Each of us has had the experience of overthinking a skill or movement by focusing on the many aspects of technique needed for performance. However, when we perform in a flow state, we are able to move holistically as one piece; as something beyond the sum of these parts.

How much time and emphasis should be spent on technique versus "yoga"? Does this vary in different contexts (classes, workshops, trainings, masterclasses)? How can you encourage students to achieve flow while applying technique?

3.7 THE MOMENT OF DEATH

Stetson, Fiesta, and Eagleman (2007) sought to understand the "feeling" of time standing still during episodes of intense fear. They created a number of experiments to see if their graduate students actually had slowed down the experience of time when "seeing their life flash before their eyes". After finding the appropriate fear-inducing event and fitting students with an apparatus to see seconds ticking off before their eyes, the data yielded interesting conclusions. Rather than time actually moving more slowly, there was a sudden opening of all the senses. The overwhelming need to process masses of sensory information created the "sense" that time had stopped, but the reality was that it continued to move along unaltered.

How does this phenomenon relate to yoga practice? How might we consciously accomplish this holistic sensorial experience without having to endanger ourselves? How would you teach it to your students?

3.8 AFFECT: NOT AFFECTATION

A teacher often suggests the assumption of qualities or mindsets as a stimulus to exploration. "What if you were to pretend your arms are very heavy?", "What if you assumed an attitude of great confidence?", "What if you were to dedicate your practice to someone you love?" The student then affects to take on these qualities – not because they arise spontaneously (though they might), but at the instigation of a suggestion. Though the word "affectation" has taken on connotations of something that is "inauthentic", the exploration of movement through the application of "affects" allows for experimentation with a high degree of personal creative investment by the student.

How might you use these cues to effectively teach?

3.9 THE LANGUAGE OF BREATH

A student's breath may reveal to what degree they perceive the unification of mind and body. Are they keeping a steady, metered breath? Are they linking breath and movement in a way that might facilitate greater knowledge of their internal state? Does the inability to maintain a steady breath indicate agitation?

Observe your own breath in practice for one week and make a detailed analysis. How does altering your breathing change your practice experience: slow, fast, metered, uneven, *kapalabhati*, alternate nostril, breath holding, nose versus mouth? Observing affect is different from observing a "postural" shape and its "correctness". It allows the teacher to speculate about how a student is experiencing their practice. In teaching, what do you notice as you focus on your students' breathing and comportment?

3.10 LEADING THE WITNESS: THE EFFECTS OF *ASANA* AND *VINYASA*

When making "suggestions" to students, expectation can skew results. If you believe that balancing while making unusual shapes with your body brings spiritual insight, enhanced emotional well-being, or better physical health, then it may very well happen. Your belief, however, should be able to account for why it may or may not happen to acrobats or contortionists. The acceptance of unsubstantiated theories may bring results that give solace if that is what is sought. In yoga classes and within parts of like communities, it is not unusual to hear ideas like the universe "has a plan" or "only gives you what you can handle", and even more specific claims such as "emotional release" after stretching of the hips. If there is an acceptance of fate or emotional release, did this happen because the student believed it was supposed to occur or was it the result of a biomechanical process?

What are examples of leading the student that you have heard or used? All teaching requires manipulation, but what kinds of manipulation are counterproductive? Does "suggesting" outcomes in instruction take away from the discriminative and exploratory skill building of the student?

3.11 PROPS AS TRAINING WHEELS

Props are utilised for the purpose of teaching. They help a student to understand what is necessary to accomplish a posture or movement and have a variety of creative uses. Props should be used thoughtfully so that they do not become objects of dependence (crutches). They are temporary measures and creative aids for teaching. During online classes, students often "create" props out of everyday objects (sofa, book, pillow, chair, belt).

How have you used props creatively in your practice and teaching? Does the same prop work for every student? How do you teach with props while fostering independence from them? When should a prop be put aside and why? How might the use of "the wall" both help and hinder learning in inversions and backbends?

3.12 OUT OF SCOPE

Students will frequently ask questions or seek advice from their teachers about problems that are tangential or unrelated to yoga. It is presumptuous for yoga teachers to assume that their knowledge of yoga gives them the answers to all life's questions.

What are you qualified to teach or advise? How do you respond when you are questioned about something for which you have no clear answer? Do you feel pressure to be an adviser for your students' life choices outside of the studio? How do you thoughtfully answer students while maintaining your role as a *yoga* teacher in order to return the responsibility for inquiry to the student?

References

Austin, James. "Effortless attention." In *A new perspective in the cognitive science of attention and action*, edited by Brian Bruya, 373–407. Cambridge, MA: Bradford, 2010.

Bartenieff, I. *Body movement: coping with the environment, identity and modernity*. Langhorne: Gordon and Breach, 1980.

Bender, Courtney. *The new metaphysicals*. Chicago: University of Chicago Press, 2010.

Calter, Paul. *Squaring the circle: geometry in art and architecture*. Hoboken: Wiley, 2008.

Clark, Bernie and Sarah Powers. *The complete guide to Yin Yoga: the philosophy and practice of Yin Yoga*. Plano: Wild Strawberry Productions, 2012.

Csikszentmihalyi, Mihaly. *Flow: the psychology of optimal experience*. New York: Harper and Row, 1990.

De Michelis, Elizabeth. *History of modern yoga*. New York: Continuum, 2005.

Durkheim, Emile. 2008. *The elementary forms of religious life*, translated by Carol Cosman. Oxford World's Classics. London: Oxford University Press.

Foxen, Anya. *Inhaling spirit: Harmonialism, Orientalism, and the Western roots of modern yoga*. Oxford: Oxford University Press, 2020.

Grilley, Paul. *Yin Yoga: principles and practice*. Ashland: White Cloud Press, 2012.

Iyengar, B.K.S. *Light on yoga*. New York: Schocken Books, 1966.

Jain, Andrea. *Selling yoga: from counterculture to pop culture*. Oxford: Oxford University Press, 2014.

Janis, Irving. "Groupthink," *Psychology Today* vol. 5 no. 6 (April, 2010): 43–46.

Jois, Sri K. Pattabhi. *Yoga Mala*. New York: North Point Press, 2010.

Mallinson, James and Mark Singleton. Roots of yoga. New York: Penguin Books, 2017.

McGilchrist, Iain. *The master and his emissary: the divided brain and the making of the Western world*. New Haven: Yale University Press, 2009.

Merleau-Ponty, M. *Phenomenology of perception*. Translated by Colin Smith. New York: Routledge and Kegan Paul, 2002: 66–68.

Metcalf, Peter. *Celebrations of death*. Cambridge: Cambridge University Press, 1992.

Nevrin, Klaus. "Empowerment and using the body in modern postural yoga." In *Yoga in the modern world*, edited by Mark Singleton and Jean Byrne, 2008: 123. London: Routledge.

Orwell, George. 1984. London: Secker and Warburg, 1949.

Sakuta, Aska. "Embodied consciousness during meditation in movement: neurocognitive theories." Extended abstract of doctoral thesis. Chichester: University of Chichester, 2017. Accessed 10 October, 2020. http://moco17.movementcomputing.org/wpcontent/uploads/2017/12/ds1-sakuta.pdf.

Sheets-Johnstone, Maxine. *The primacy of movement*. Amsterdam: Johns Benjamins, 1999.

Sheets-Johnstone, Maxine. "Why is movement therapeutic?" *American Journal of Dance Therapy* vol. 32 no. 1 (2010): 2–15.

Singleton, Mark. *Yoga body: the origins of modern posture practice*. Oxford: Oxford University Press, 2010.

Smith, M.I. "Moving Self: the thread which bridges dance and theatre." *Research in Dance Education*, vol. 3 no. 2 (2002).

Stetson, C., M.P. Fiesta, D.M. Eagleman. "Does time really slow down during a frightening event?" PLoS ONE (2007): vol. 2 no. 12: e1295. Accessed 3 April, 2020. https://doi.org/10.1371/journal.pone.0001295

Sweeney, R. *Transferring principles: the role of physical consciousness in Butoh and its application within contemporary performance praxis*. London: Middlesex University, 2009.

Whyte, Jr., "Groupthink." *Fortune*, 1952. Accessed 3 April, 2020. https://fortune.com/2012/07/22/groupthink-fortune-1952/.

Wilkerson, Abby. *Embodiment*. New York: New York University Press, 2015. Accessed 12 April, 2020. https://doi.org/10.18574/9781479812141-022.

Zarelli, Phillip. "Toward a phenomenological model of the actor's embodied modes of experience." *Theatre Journal*, vol. 56 (2004): 653–666.

Zink, Paulie and Maria March. "Yin Yoga." *Yoga Magazine* (2012).

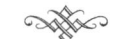

Chapter Four
The Business of Yoga
To Teach or Not to Teach

THE BOOMING FIELD OF YOGA EDUCATION

Yoga has certainly succeeded in becoming a fixture in popular culture around the world, enjoying a reputation as a global phenomenon. The reasons for yoga's popularity are complex, but as Andrea Jain notes in *Selling Yoga*, free market capitalism, the increased ability for people and ideas to travel to disparate parts of the world, "widespread disillusionment with established religious traditions," and the "merging with global consumer culture" have supported the global popularisation of yoga (Jain 2015, 43). With popularity has come the proliferation of teacher training programmes and an ever-increasing number of people who desire to train as teachers. Not everyone who takes teacher training ends up teaching yoga; many never intend to teach yoga at all. What accounts for this phenomenon and why are teacher training programmes so popular?

While yoga is undeniably popular, there are problems with the modern business model that most studios follow. Rather than adopt a school model, studios have become more like gyms. Classes are provided at accessible times for the convenience of their clientele often to the detriment of the progressive instruction that could be delivered in courses. The advancement of students through a curriculum is largely disregarded

DOI: 10.4324/9781003181910-5

because the necessity to pay rent, retain popular teachers, and stay current with trends takes precedence. As will be discussed further, this leads many novice practitioners to enrol in teacher training to advance their practice without the requisite foundational knowledge or experience. To accommodate this, many studios have low or few standards, both for application and completion of teacher training.

YOGA AS POPULAR CULTURE

As Jain describes, in the last half of the twentieth century, yoga became firmly fixed within popular culture. As the masses made and continue to make "choices" about what to consume, they created pop culture through this very act of consumption (Jain 2015, 45), in particular in urban areas around the world. Modern yogis are no longer the subject of suspicion and censorship, as they were in the past (the purveyors of esoteric, marginal, or countercultural practices). Instead, yoga enjoys positive press as a body regimen that improves health and well-being for the masses (Jain 2015, 46). What made yoga attractive to many was that it was disengaged from any religious tradition or belief system (although this is still a point of contestation by Hindu nationalist groups like HAF)[1] and that it promised to solve a wide variety of social, psychological, and spiritual ills of modern life. As Courtney Bender notes in her ethnographic work, *The New Metaphysicals*, once detached from its overtly religious associations, yoga connected itself to a number of Western institutional contexts, through which it found its meaning and authenticity. Newly understood as "spirituality", it comes to mean for those who practice it something distinctly different from "religion". As Bender notes of many modern metaphysical traditions like yoga:

> …what organizes spirituality appears to be a "market" and a choice, where each individual consumer and seeker confronts a marketplace of undifferentiated and changing goods…what we think of as the spiritual is actively produced within medical, religious and arts institutions, among others. It is not unorganized or disorganized, but rather organized in different ways, within and adjacent to a variety of religious and secular fields that inflect and shape various spiritual practices…metaphysicals engage the spiritual in different institutional settings, including some that are usually considered secular.
>
> (Bender 2010, 22–23)

Yoga, like many other "spiritual" endeavours, has been contextualised and enacted through many institutions, most notably the healing/therapy and other allied medical fields, fitness, and health industries, as stress reduction and parapsychology, and as "community" in social and political milieus. It is not that these associations are fallacious, but that they have implications that are often left largely unaddressed and unexamined both by practitioners and yoga organisations.

For example, when yoga aligns itself with the medical profession, it is subject to the standards, evaluations, and restrictions of medical organisations and medical institutions. Yoga in this context is both validated by and dependent upon the results of medical studies and healing testimonials. This has led to the increasing regulation and codification of yoga through newly formed yoga therapy organisations like the IAYT and SYTAR.[2] By identifying as healers (whether certified or not), teachers now attract students who are in a state of "disease" and seeking relief. This raises questions about whether teachers are aware of the responsibility of their role as healers or prepared for students who may be in a heightened state of "need". If unaware of these issues, teachers may be placing themselves in a vulnerable position, where students have expectations of them that they cannot – or are ill-prepared – to fill. Positioning oneself as a healer has a multitude of repercussions, not the least of which is that the exactitude of medical standards for efficacy may preclude yoga's broader spiritual aspirations.

Within mental health contexts, yoga is believed to be beneficial in treating everything from everyday stress to deeply somaticised trauma. In this milieu, the language of yoga reflects the worldview of the mental health community. This alignment has led to the creation of a variety of yoga intervention systems that function within the modality of mental health like "trauma sensitive yoga", "prison yoga", "wounded warriors", and "yoga for addiction". Authenticity narratives focus on redemption and healing from trauma and other psychological maladies. Validation is understood through the language of *twelve-step* and other systems of mental health remediation (Khoshaba 2013).

Beliefs about universal toxicity (acquired through one's occupation, family, relationships, diet, trauma, ecological degradation, technology) are supported by presenting yoga as a system of "therapy" – physical, psychological, or emotional. This plays on existential angst in the Western world seen in light of fears about end times, climate change, and the prevalence of conspiratorial thinking – conspiracy theories abound in the yoga community.[3] Despite the fact that yoga may align itself with Western medicine and thereby science, there persists a coexistent, yet anomalous, belief that biomedicine is not to be trusted. Rather, many prefer to believe ancient Ayurvedic medicine (or other natural systems of healing) to be a superior system, despite most yoga practitioners' limited knowledge or interaction with it.

Within the fitness industry, yoga functions as a physical regimen to build strength and flexibility, which has spawned many fitness-yoga hybrids like YogaFit, Pycor, Yogalates, and other systems that subsume the socio-spiritual aspects of practice and incorporate both the language (core strength) and standards of the fitness industry. Part of the initial reluctance to practice yoga in the Western milieu was because yoga was viewed as a "religion". Aligned with fitness, yoga becomes more easily consumed, and must promote the safety and healthfulness of practice. This encourages both regulation and standardisation to lessen liability.[4] Fitness narratives stress the superiority of yoga as a system for physical conditioning, attractiveness, and even anti-ageing. The focus on physical appearance as a marker of fitness has resulted in the common occurrence of eating disorders among practitioners (especially women) who desire the ideal "yoga body",[5] and an inaccurate perception of the way that yoga is capable of transforming every *body*. A quick search through magazine articles online tout yoga as a miracle for body sculpting; promising "lean muscles" (not bulky or masculine), "slim and fit frame", and "better sex life". In fact, part of the reforms currently espoused in yoga call for a change to a "body positive" rather than a "body beautiful" emphasis in strong opposition to this focus. As Kimberly Dark notes on the site *Decolonizing Yoga*:

> It's inevitable in a consumer culture that the people who can afford to pay a yoga teacher what she's worth will be interested in status. And "hot body" definitely equates status. Sometimes the noble fat person can sneak through – the beginner who's assumed to be fighting the good fight against her or his own flab. That person can be jovially accommodated and feel a little bit of love. But what of the average plodder who does a regular practice and never *looks* [sic] fit? Well, sometimes it's just not comfortable, so the group support and individual instruction offered by beautiful studios are forfeit. Even if the fat yogi persists through the initial discomfort and becomes a regular, the feeling of being an outsider can persist.
>
> (Dark 2014)

Yoga merchandising relies on the selling of slim, fit, and sexy bodies. In Western culture, "physical attractiveness" is equated with appearance, especially for women. The conflation of bodily appearance and fitness is not unique to yoga. However, the degree to which women's bodies (as athletes) are judged by appearance and normative sexuality is marked in yoga – so much so, that "fat" or "sexually unappealing" women may not even feel welcome in the practice at all. As San Francisco yoga teacher Kimber Simpkins noted of the dearth of queer women in yoga compared to other fitness activities: "It's important that we work to undo that negative internalisation because otherwise, we can unconsciously believe that our discomfort is our own fault and that we have to change our bodies to fix it. Just as we work hard to let go of society's expectations about who we should love, we have to let go of society's expectations around what we should look like" (Curtis 2018).

As Bender notes, some yoga practitioners align themselves with religious rather than secular institutions. Yoga classes have long been held in the basements of churches and in YMCAs. In this context, yoga takes on a spiritual character, and the physical practice is diminished in importance. Yoga is accepted alongside other religious beliefs as a complimentary practice or hybridised in religion-specific systems. *Christian Yoga* arose as a way to ensure that Jesus remains the focus of spiritual engagement, but, more likely, the religious aspects of yoga are tamed through denuding the status or power of the teacher. "Americans are comfortable with yoga as a non-religious physical endeavour. It is acceptable when portrayed through the homespun, educated and refreshingly freethinking, familiar girl next door. If we didn't homogenise the face of yoga this way, yoga in America would be a closet activity, deemed inappropriate for Christians" (Lawson 2013). Within religious institutional contexts, yoga is reframed as a transformational and mystical (one that connects the participant directly to "God") technique, where meditation (spiritual) or prayer (religious) are valued as the principal goals of yoga practice.

Another outcome of the alignment of yoga with religion is the evolution of a set of ethics that prescribe an ideal lifestyle. Yoga was traditionally ethically neutral; since all is formed from the same energy or all an expression of supreme consciousness, the "yogi is [both] god, and the yogi is the devil" (Fouce 2005). One critique of the *Bhagavad Gita* is that it lacks ethical prescriptions and instead promotes an extreme sort of moral relativism (Wayne 2017). More recently, yoga was contextually aligned with the countercultural movement and a rejection of conventional norms for behaviour. Today, there is a shift in alignment toward liberal and progressive ideals. Yoga is now firmly aligned, both in the public imagination and among practitioners, with ethical practice, one that demands yoga practitioners and teachers hold certain political positions and subscribe to a set of beliefs. The *yamas* and *niyamas* are heightened in importance and brought out as exemplars of required beliefs and comportment, but there is nothing uniquely yogic about them, nor anything essential in them for the performance of somatic practice. In general, modern yoga "ethics" serve to restrict behaviour rather than encourage the abandonment of social stricture in the service of self-exploration.

In addition to religious texts, Bender speaks of the importance of "experiential texts" in the personal and social validation of the mystical practitioners she studied. Within each story, she identified three tropes that help to form authoritative narratives: "modes of temporal unfolding, the description of social ties within the plot, and the assertion of embodied or emotional knowledge over cognitive knowledge" (Bender 2010, 62). Here, important (embodied) feelings and emotions become powerful markers of authenticity that trump both institutional authority and facts. This amplifies the believability of experiential personal texts as authoritative documents, even in the face of contradicting evidence (science).

The Ideal of "Community"

Modern yoga's most profound contextual alignment is with the notion of *community*. For yoga practitioners, community has many aspects. It refers to the strong bonds, like-mindedness, and allegiance that practitioners have to their local studio. It more broadly refers to the world yoga community, and, furthermore, the universal connectedness of pure consciousness. Community has become ubiquitous, as is seen in yoga merchandising, trade journals, and discussion about the yogic lifestyle. The notion of community, like the notion of *friendship*, has been significantly transformed in the age of social media. On the one hand, technology allows one to connect with others in ways never before possible. On the other hand, these relationships have become diminished through their expansion. In fact, despite the increased opportunities for connection, people generally express higher levels of detachment and separation.

Facebook, Twitter and an almost fully-connected world of the Internet, computers, smartphones and cell phones have surely changed how people relate to the world around them and how they feel about themselves. Some wired people feel reassured that they are part of an ever-larger, albeit synthetic, crowd of friends. Others strangely feel lonelier as they imagine that the legions of people they are connected to do not really "get" them.

(Agnew and Brezina 2010, 134)

Long before social media, French sociologist Emile Durkheim gave a name to this kind of crowd loneliness – *anomie*; the state of mind describing disaffected people who are more than normally susceptible to being misled by misguided people. With today's proliferation of "friends", things become seriously distorted; instead of old-fashioned anomie, today people are experiencing magnification of their sensibilities both positively and negatively. This distortion can leave many beholden to and dependent upon their "community" or teachers, in ways that are neither satisfying nor healthy. The sense of belonging associated with the creation and nurturing of community is particularly sought after by yoga practitioners, but the need for belonging and the marked expectations placed on community leaders may result in an equally marked sense of disillusionment amongst community members who feel unsatisfied or unnoticed.

In her published dissertation, Theodora Wildcroft looks at "post-lineage yoga" as a new movement of devoted practitioners, formed in opposition to modern transnational orthodox practices. As she states, "Post-lineage yoga is a re-evaluation of the authority to determine practice, and a privileging of peer networks over pedagogical hierarchies, or *sanghas* (communities) over *guru-śiṣya* (teacher-adept) relationships" (Wildcroft 2018a, 15). Post-lineage yogis are a group of dedicated practitioners, most of whom are disillusioned by modern lineage organisations and patriarchal power structures, who see themselves as a democratic, inclusive, and equalitarian practice community. This diffuse community comes together at a series of yearly festivals in various parts of the world to codify, validate, and practice their shared system of beliefs and behaviours. In this sense, the community itself has become the force of authority, and the community members, the source of validation. Though not all modern practitioners identify with post-lineal values and beliefs,[6] many studios share this valourisation and empowerment of community. This has resulted in the diminishment of the authority and perceived superior skill or knowledge of the teacher in many studio settings; that authority now rests on the collective judgements of the community itself. In such contexts, external validation by the teacher has been replaced by the necessity for external validation by the practice community, whose strictures may be just as curtailed as the *guru's* once were. In some yoga systems, veganism isn't a dietary option, it is a moral requirement that is preached in class. Likewise, environmentalism, anti-colonialism, and other progressive political beliefs are expected of those who practice yoga as they are seen by the community as evidence of "enlightened" thinking and practice.

The centrality of community, however narrowly or broadly defined, should not be underestimated in modern postural yoga, whether it exists inside (post-lineal yoga) or outside a formally imagined structure. Coupled with the importance of community is the institutional context, whether secular or religious, through which yoga is integrated into Western culture. It is with knowledge of these considerations that a practitioner should choose to teach, as the context and the community they choose will determine how their teaching is received. In light of this, how does the studio setting compare to the other institutionalised structures to which yoga might be aligned?

THE BUSINESS MODEL OF YOGA: ITS IMPACT ON TEACHING

Many yoga teachers and studio owners would argue that the "business of yoga" is anything but a money-making enterprise; they bemoan their lack of ability to sustain themselves or their studio space, let alone earn a living through teaching. If yoga is arguably highly commodified, as so many suggest, who is getting rich selling the product being marketed? Many studios find that financial viability comes through anything but yoga classes. Yoga products, coffee and tea bars, body work, a variety of healing modalities, and alternative practices abound – they are selling things that are ancillary to yoga (happiness, health, meaning, purpose, sex appeal, community).

When the modern conception of a yoga studio was first adopted, few would have predicted that it would profoundly influence the way yoga is taught and that these changes were potentially malign. Before the advent of dedicated yoga studios, physical yoga classes were, as often as not, weekly sessions held in rented spaces (community halls, church basements) that served a variety of purposes. The classes teachers gave were homespun labours-of-love and served a diversity of levels. If the teacher needed a substitute, one of the senior students would fill in. The profession of yoga teacher did not exist. Students' progress was a slow, but cumulative, process for those who kept at it. The dedicated yoga studio led to swifter advancement of students' physical skills, particularly in the range of hand balances and inversions,[7] because more classes meant people had the opportunity to practice more often. Such rapid and palpable learning of unusual balances and other postures gave bright prospects for the success of yoga studios. While initially studios were the vision of one teacher in particular, the practicalities of the number of classes an individual teacher had to give weekly for such premises to function financially meant that it was necessary to engage other teachers. In establishing their own dedicated premises, most studios adopted business models and practices found in the gym and fitness industries.

The most marked similarity between gyms and yoga studios is the way they schedule classes. So pervasive is this template that it can be difficult to see what effect it has had. The schedule lays out a selection of classes for the week. Classes are held at regular times and have set time limits. Typically, there are early morning, lunchtime, and evening classes because these are the times that are easiest for attendees with jobs and families to accommodate. Most classes are intended for a "general" level, though yoga studios may offer more "advanced" level classes than gyms. The levels set out by individual studios (and gyms) are arbitrary and case specific. In practice, a teacher might find themselves giving a Level 1 (a designation that would vary from studio to studio) class on Monday, Wednesday, and Friday at 6:00 PM. This is potentially demoralising for the teacher. There is no guarantee that they will be teaching the same people on each of these days, nor from week to week. They may have a regular client base who become familiar with what they teach, but it is also incumbent on them to accommodate newcomers and it is in the studio's interest to encourage an influx of new students. This means that gyms and yoga studios will always hold more low-level classes. Because the timing of classes is made to suit the client's convenience, it is difficult to move most people on to more advanced levels. If people are happy with the schedule, they have no incentive to move to a class where they may feel the frustration of challenges. In the gym model, it is paramount that the client feels happy with their experience; if not, they may take their business elsewhere.

It is hard to argue with an ethos of keeping people happy while they move their bodies, but the level at which they are capable of doing so varies. If everyone is welcome in yoga, what criteria does a studio establish for turning people away from a class that is too advanced for them? Surely, an accomplished teacher should be able to facilitate a "happy" experience for beginners, intermediate, and advanced students in the same room. However, a supervisory role of the less advanced usually comes with this and this comes at the expense of development of the more advanced. More novice students require attention and supervision from the teacher to ensure that they understand the instructions and are safe from injury. But, because many studios are financially challenged, it is a luxury to turn lower-level students away even though admission to the class is ethically questionable however much one wants to adhere to making yoga accessible for all.

When yoga becomes a business, yoga teachers face further unpalatable realities. They will have to teach a lot of classes to make a living. They will likely have to travel between several studios to do so. There are further problems for a teacher's financial solvency: studio rivalries may be such that they are asked not to teach at other studios and be required to commit to exclusivity. As class times are scheduled in the early morning and in the evening, yoga teachers' employment often requires them to teach during both slots. This may be fine to do for a few weeks, but the yoga studio schedule is relentless – it goes for 52 weeks per year.

In the past, class lengths were open ended and at the discretion of the teacher. This allowed for the teacher to continue until the class reached an organic conclusion. Though teachers can configure classes within set time constraints, there is no possibility for the teacher to continue teaching when there are students at the door waiting for the next class. The exigencies of the client getting what they paid for takes precedence over educational imperatives.

However, there are significant differences between gyms and yoga studios. Gyms are more heavily invested in equipment and people use them on an ad hoc basis at any time they like – some remaining open 24 hours a day. Gym facilities make large investment in showers, towels, and changing rooms while yoga studios, as often as not, make do with curtains and a toilet with a sink. Classes at gyms are various and quite often are included in membership fees or at least at a cost below what yoga studios find necessary to charge. Many studios attempt to attract students with deals such as "90 days for $90" while acknowledging (like gym memberships) that many taking advantage of such offers do not regularly pursue them for the duration. If so, it is important to ensure that the studio's marketing is sufficiently effective at finding new prospects to maintain revenue flow. If there is a strong emphasis on attracting newcomers to the studio, there is also emphasis on developing the clientele. Yoga studios are able to outperform gyms in this regard; the ethos of a gym class is on participation, not education – less time is spent on refining and analysing technique. The philosophy of gyms is geared towards healthfulness through activity. Yoga is well adapted to this as a philosophy too, but it does add a strong dose of spirituality. For some, this is not appealing and would be a contributing factor to ultimately choosing a gym over a studio. As the major emphasis is on newcomers, the discernment of the clientele is not necessarily well informed as to the quality of teaching. Before yoga classes became a staple of gyms, they already ran successful versions of aerobic exercise in the prime-time slots and, when yoga was first introduced, it was relegated to less popular times. Most yoga studios can only hold profitable classes for four or five hours a day. Some try to fill the "dead" times with specialised classes (pre- and post-natal, moms and tots) and occasional weekend workshops. Of these, the workshops are usually the more profitable, but less regular. They are "special" and holding them too often lessens their novelty. The most successful schedule filler has been teacher training. A rationale for teacher training is that it produces revenue flow and can be done at times when the space is not being used. Teacher training is not driven by a need for more teachers, but by a lack of students.

The Teacher Training Industry

The difficulty in sustaining a studio space is marked, but the benefits to having a separate yoga space are important as well. Acknowledging the influence that institutional alignment has on restricting the interpretation and authority of teachers and their offerings, a studio provides a separate space where yogis can structure alternative values, beliefs, and practices adjacent to these institutions. In short, yoga practiced in a studio setting has the potential to enjoy greater independence from the aforementioned institutional structures outlined by Bender. Simply having a studio space does not disjoin yoga practice from hegemonic culture; it does, however, offer the opportunity for a degree of independence from it.

The independence found in studio settings poses difficulties; among them, how to sell a *vision* without appearing to be a business; for yoga teachers are expected to do their teaching "out of service and out of love". This has, in part, led to the explosion of yoga teacher training programmes in the West, along with yoga retreats and specialised modalities, for which secondary training is developed and sold. Fuelling this fire was the development spearheaded by the Yoga Alliance of the 200-hour teacher training, and 300 (nee 500) hour advanced training. Once "advanced" certification became established, an "experienced" teacher could begin running training at an average cost of $3000 per person. Many such teacher training courses require no prerequisites, making the rejection of applications unlikely. Ancillary and advanced training, and a proliferation of additional certifications and shadowing programmes, provided a welcome respite for studios trying to make ends meet. The "degree inflation" in yoga is illustrated by the number of letters and numbers following practitioners' names, which carry little meaning. This system replaced the more traditional systems that required long-served mentorship with a teacher who ensured that their charges were well-prepared to teach. Today, teacher training programmes are often less protracted (for the convenience of trainees and studios) and require comparatively little or no continual in-depth study with a knowledgeable practitioner. This has resulted in a glut of ill-prepared teachers, many of whom do not have prerequisite skills in practicing yoga, nor any substantial knowledge of the discipline. As one yoga teacher said of their own studio, "pretty soon, everyone at my place will be a certified yoga teacher...what then?" Recognising this, Yoga Alliance has responded by "elevating" its standards, requiring higher levels of expertise for "lead teachers", and expanded content categories to "promote high quality, safe, accessible, and equitable yoga teaching" – and training (Yoga Alliance, 2020). Whether these changes will resolve these issues remains to be seen since the diminished duration of training has not been addressed, especially in light of the "expanded content".

As Bender would certainly note, aligning one's discipline with a codifying institution makes gaining validity subject to the values, beliefs, and strictures of that organisation (Yoga Alliance). Started in 1999 in the United States, Yoga Alliance has grown to influence yoga studios worldwide. Yoga Alliance does not certify teachers; they are a registry that individual teachers and schools may join to have their services marketed. As such, Yoga Alliance is part of the yoga industry; a component of the studio/gym business model. It is a professional organisation providing credentials for participation in the business of yoga. The requirements for membership are bureaucratic and financial, as Yoga Alliance does not directly evaluate or oversee the quality of teachers or programmes. Membership requirements for Yoga Alliance are inclusive because it is more important that they stand as a "community of inclusion" rather than a place of excellence. Consequently, there exists an industry that has failed to guarantee the quality of their members, many of whom have gone on to train subsequent generations of teachers. Yoga Alliance has tried to address these deficits, proposing an overhaul of the standards and a reworking of the credentialling process.

Some lineages and schools do not participate in Yoga Alliance. Ashtanga, Iyengar, and Bikram have their own certification systems, which are rigorous and highly scrutinised with clear oversight. They do not require Yoga Alliance registration (although some teachers may choose to join for marketing purposes) since their credentials are standardised and unquestioned. People who are not sanctioned by an orthodoxy find themselves in need of the Yoga Alliance for marketing and the appearance of legitimacy. This has created animosity between the Yoga Alliance and some yoga teachers.

The proliferation of teacher training resulted in a glut of teachers and continues to exert a profound impact on the development of yoga as a discipline. This includes competition for teaching positions and students, the inability for students to recognise, vet, or find quality teachers, and the lack of tools that aspiring teachers are given to assess yoga training programmes. An additional impact may be the reported high rate for injuries in yoga. According to a 2017 study published in *Science Daily*, "Yoga causes musculoskeletal pain in 10 percent of people and exacerbates 21 percent of existing injuries … The findings come from the first prospective study to investigate injuries caused from recreational participation in yoga. The injury rate is up to 10 times higher than has previously been reported" (University of Sydney 2017). Such findings may also account for a general diminution of and respect for the discipline of yoga and its practitioners.

The adoption of the business model of yoga has led to a shift in the way yoga studios view those who come to practice; they have become clients rather than students. This shift is significant: while students are taught what the teacher deems important according to the rigours of the discipline, there is pressure to give clients what *they* want – clients have paid admission and studios' survival is dependent on retaining them. Despite the espousal of "community", competition between studios for clients has compounded this problem. The lack of cooperation between studios and lack of encouragement to explore other modes of practice or other teachers beyond the home studio is decidedly in the service of studio survival and not the students themselves. This further curtails the evolution and vibrancy of the discipline as well as the students' progress. Competition for business has also led to some studio models that offer donation or low-cost classes. This often results in large classes where personalised and responsive teaching is difficult, and emphasis is framed around broad and inclusive access to studio classes to maintain a client base.

Why Teach?

Why would one want to be a teacher? If one has achieved a high level of experience and competency in practice, they may desire to share their accumulated knowledge with others. Those who have experienced great mentoring and inspiration from their teachers may wish to pass down this knowledge as a way of honouring that legacy. However, people increasingly embark on training programmes with insufficient practice experience or knowledge. This is bolstered by a studio system that promotes teacher training as a way to sustain financial solvency and encourages clients to maintain membership in the studio community. Teacher training functions as a way to become part of the "tribe" and community membership is not solidified until the training is completed. Novice teachers become initiates to the studio elite; a status to which they aspire. For the studio, this satisfies the need for continued financial support and, for the novice teacher, a sense of higher status and belonging.

Teaching is also a way to better understand a discipline, a sentiment frequently expressed in the adage, "you don't really know something until you teach it". The process of breaking down yoga concepts and techniques so that they are "teachable" demands that one critically examine their understanding of the material so it can be articulated clearly. The idea that one learns through the teaching (and training) process is often used as a way to encourage inexperienced students to take teacher training. Many students say they do not know if they want to teach but view teacher training as a way to learn yoga – in a way they cannot in studio classes. But why can't they find and take "better" classes rather than expensive teacher training? A dearth of progressive or intensive courses forces students to seek out either private instruction or teacher training. Studio solvency requires that clients invest in these expensive options and, to encourage this, may offer more limited instruction during regular classes. This may indicate a failure of the studio model, or just a reality of the commodification of yoga; the making of a yoga industry rather than a practical vocation.

Some practitioners choose to leave lucrative, but highly stressful, jobs, to take teacher training because they aspire to do something "meaningful" – something they cannot achieve in their workaday life. Others feel that yoga teaching is a spiritual calling. Many who work in the self-help and self-care industries see yoga certification and teaching as a useful adjunct to their metaphysical, holistic, or life coach training and pursue licensure as a way to add to their credentials. Though these are admirable intentions, a teacher's success depends on the quality and depth of the training undertaken and their ability to apply their skills and knowledge in practice.

"Anyone Can Do Yoga!"

Though the *guru* is much revered in the East, the vocation of teaching is both respected and *contested* in Western culture. Once an honourable and much-admired profession, the status of teacher (not solely in yoga) is, in many ways, diminished and the teacher's authority subject to question. In such an environment, being a successful teacher is a challenging enterprise. Teachers are often maligned as to their capabilities; the quip "those who can't do, teach" speaks to this lack of respect; the insinuation being that one who teaches has failed in the profession they instruct. Teachers in the West are expected to deliver information and are responsible for their students' successful learning. The student who fails to learn is largely free from responsibility and the teacher is reduced to the mechanism for the delivery of a product: a certification, a degree, a grade.

In addition, there is the notion in yoga that "anyone can do yoga". Though this sentiment is meant to encourage everyone to practise and to emphasise the individualised nature of yoga as a somatic enterprise, it has resulted, in many cases, in the belief that students "are perfect the way they are" and therefore do not need correction. Rather, what they need is more akin to "coaching" or simply encouragement; for, if the student is perfect in their individual expression, what right does the teacher have to make a correction? This is bolstered by a larger movement in Western culture that may be referred to as the "no judgment culture credo", where passing judgement has become synonymous with ignorance or a biased perspective. Corrections are viewed as a failure to accept the "different" way that students might "correctly" express themselves in practice – as judgemental attitudes.

It is the perspective herein that each expression of somatic practice is unique and that *standards* based on the teacher's theory, method, and techniques provide a foundation for critique. In essence, there are many "right" ways to execute a yoga practice, and also some that are wrong. For example, students will often ask, "does it matter if I put my arm here, instead of here?" The answer is always "yes"; everything matters. It is essential to distinguish what variations are *not* possible within the context of the system in which one experiments. For instance, in some theories of breath and movement, to kick up into a handstand is incorrect, if breath is understood as the basis of movement. It isn't that one cannot get up by kicking up, but that it violates the premise of the theory – and the method and techniques aligned with it. But how can a teacher express this in a climate where critique is seen as judgement? Teachers explain their corrections in terms of theory and method and supply a route to improvement that is clear and consistent.

Everyone Is a Teacher

If anyone can do yoga, then why can't everyone train to teach? In many cases, everyone can, regardless of their experience, skill set, knowledge, or ability. Beginners may be told they would make "a great teacher", and that taking teacher training is an excellent way to learn yoga. The justification of using training as a way to learn yoga fails to recognise that learning to do yoga and teaching yoga are different skills and enterprises.

All You Need Is Love

Aspiring teachers of yoga may be told that one cannot learn how to teach (that this skill arises naturally), and instead be encouraged to "love" yoga, which becomes the principal goal of training. The idea is that, out of love for yoga, there will arise a passion for teaching (although the skill set on the subject may be absent). So, is to "love" yoga and have good intentions enough, and what is this love? Is it a profound interest in the subject? Does it mean that yoga gives one joy (the promised bliss)? Or is it mere infatuation – the intensity of experience that one generally enjoys when making new discoveries? Does one need to understand something to actually love it? If this passion is enough, how might it be sustained? Does sustaining passion require dedication and discipline?

SUSTAINING A TEACHING VOCATION

How can one sustain their passion for yoga, and what does one do to "keep at it" when that passion inevitably ebbs and flows? The day to day of teaching is not filled with passionate moments. More likely, it is filled with repetition. It is important to sustain a strong, personal practice – to make time for one's own exploration, study, and advancement to inspire their teaching. This can be challenging because teaching frequent classes is fatiguing, and, concomitantly, because teachers lack the time to devote to their personal enrichment. To this end, teachers who want to avoid burnout should think about scheduling quite critically. Students may want their teachers to teach more or schedule times that work for them, but teachers need to remember that their teaching begins with their own adequate preparation and support. Failure to find time and the means to do this will make one less apt to maintain excellence or enjoyment in teaching.

It is both satisfying and empowering to watch students advance. Many practitioners begin teaching and are sustained by the positive feeling they receive in watching others successfully achieve their goals. This is usually supported by a propensity to enjoy problem-solving (either the teacher's or the student's), since every challenge may be viewed as a conundrum to solve. The problem-solving perspective helps sustain interest in both teaching and personal exploration. Analysis of one's own practice may occur while teaching and this may also serve to inspire or maintain interest. Finally, teachers may enter the profession to make money and, if successful, this certainly sustains their interest.

Why Do People Stop Teaching?

People leave teaching for a number of reasons. Teachers may be disillusioned if they fail to attract students to their classes. This is particularly the case if the studio encourages teaching quotas or pays teachers on commission, or the money made in teaching is unsustainable. A lack of inspiration, burn out, or injury are also common reasons why some leave the teaching profession. If a teacher opens a studio, they may find that their administrative responsibilities leave no time for teaching, practice, or other personal obligations. Those who have other employment that supplements their work as yoga teachers may struggle with the time and effort necessary to sustain both careers and opt to give up teaching. Finally, some stop teaching because they simply find they do not enjoy it.

Inspiration and interest ultimately arise from within the teacher. Any situation is potent with opportunity. Small classes are occasions to practice pedagogical skills, even though they may lack the motivation of financial reward or energetic excitement found in larger classes. With a small class, one has more time to observe and adjust students and create a deeper learning experience than a larger class allows. Teachers can also use small classes to hone their skills in teaching private or small groups. Here, the focus of instruction is adapted to the needs of the students who are present. Teachers should recognise that good teaching is not dependent on who or how many students attend their classes. They are inspired by their personal desire for excellence and their ability to creatively adapt to any teaching situation.

The management of time has its own challenges. Studio ownership has demands that are rarely considered by prospective owners, and one needs to be clear-eyed about it being a time-consuming job, not just a labour of love. Likewise, teaching requires hours of planning and practice outside of the time spent with students. An excess of classes eats into the time necessary for this planning and development. This can result in repetitive teaching, which may be a source of boredom or disillusionment. Teachers should be honest about how much they can do and what they can sacrifice (family, relationships, professional development, other career responsibilities) while still making teaching rewarding.

HOW DO TEACHERS, PRACTITIONERS, AND STUDENTS DIFFER?

Teaching, practicing, and learning are not the same thing. They are separate experiences that require different skills and have very different priorities. Familiarity with the challenges of learning, and having a disciplined practice of their own, are essential qualities of a good *teacher*. A teacher's empathy for students arises from these experiences. *Students* are led through a set of techniques so they can have the larger synthetic experience called "yoga" (the experience of practice). They observe the teacher and themselves, as well as others in the class, and then experiment with the information gathered. Through this process, they discover how to properly function as *practitioners.* As mentioned in Chapter 3, the best teachers present information to students in a way that they are most likely to receive and process it. The learning is the purview of the student; each student will hear and integrate information in different ways depending on many factors (e.g., level of understanding, desire for mastery, ability to listen, intensity of focus and concentration). Practitioners have absorbed through study the essential techniques and methods required to enable a "yoga" experience on their own. Teachers teach, practitioners do, and students learn.

The Experience of Teaching

The teacher is situated outside of the "here and now" experience relative to that of the student or practitioner. The teacher must observe and analyse, whereas those practicing are engaged in the experience; an action that is neither reflective nor projective. Observation necessitates separation; the teacher attends to the nuanced performance of their students to allow evaluation. This observation includes the smoothness of students' physical movements, stability, stillness, and other physical indicators of their holistic state. The analysis considers the potential of the student (immediate and future), as well as referencing the teacher's own experience of practice. This distancing makes "teaching" yoga different from "doing" yoga, where the practitioner's experience strives for a state of *flow* found in the synthesis of details gained through the analysis and observation of themselves.

Teachers must have the ability to clearly demonstrate and communicate instruction regarding physical movement and breath. When necessary, teachers must deliver clear and effective criticism and corrections and have a variety of teaching methods to accommodate different students. Teachers must manage time, so they can properly sequence and implement effective class instruction. Analysis requires multiple perspectives. The teacher cross-references their knowledge of yoga with the students' capabilities. Through observation, the teacher hones their ability to "see". The skills of analysis and observation are entwined since the teacher must "know" what they want to observe in their students, "see" what is actually occurring, and "understand" how to move students toward these goals. Finally, a teacher, through their own accomplishments, knowledge, and dedication possesses the ability to motivate and inspire their students to evolve into practitioners.

Skills and Self-Development

The skill set required for practicing yoga is a necessary foundation for teaching, but it is not enough; teachers must also develop and hone a number of additional skills. While practicing is a personal experience that requires contemplation, teaching is simultaneously the experience of inward reflection and outward observation. The dual vision that teachers need requires the development of empathy in addition to keen observational and analytical skills. Developing empathy is a difficult process, since it requires that one actually "feel" the experiences of others; it is different from sympathising or having compassion. Sympathy requires only an intellectual understanding of what someone else is experiencing, and compassion is the ability to care. To empathise with others, one must have confronted their own physical and psychological limitations. This is one reason it is so important for teachers to regularly place themselves in challenging practices, where the risk is high and the outcome uncertain. Injury, or other debilitating situations, may also be a source of empathy (although not desired), since they give one a bodily appreciation of the challenges faced by students. It is also important to understand the difficulties for those who excel at practice. Their struggles may be just as extensive, and rarely acknowledged. Many students who are flexible, for example, have difficulty balancing and holding postures that require strength. They also may lack the ability to "feel" when they overstretch or lose the necessary stability in their joints. Valourising flexibility can result in overlooking these real challenges, which often lead to a lack of progress or injury.

Expertise should necessarily be a precursor to teaching; too often the aspiration to teach arises from a desire to belong or be admired, rather than confidence in one's knowledge. A lack of expertise may lead teachers to make bad decisions about boundaries (e.g., blurring lines in relationships with students, needing to be liked by students, framing classes around students' desires rather than what is important to teach), or lead to pushing students into excessively demanding sequences (asking students to do things that are inappropriate – e.g., 50 chaturangas). A teacher who lacks the ability to do what they require of their students may not appreciate that it could be injurious or gratuitous. This insecurity may make a teacher more likely to need admiration or to seem exceptionally demanding as proof of their competency. Competent teachers convey the subtlety that comes from deep understanding; they know that what appears simple is often very difficult and that "flashy" postures are not necessarily indicative of yogic skill.

Specific competencies are necessary for teaching. A teacher understands how the body works in stillness and movement, and the physical, intellectual, and emotional demands of practice. A teacher must be able to gain, sustain, and re-establish focus and concentration, so they can convey the purpose of these techniques. The teacher must have a skilful practice, which involves the ability to integrate intention with execution. A teacher also needs to be an autodidact, to discover their own questions; a teacher's questions and interests provide a foundation for exploration. When one practises on their own, they learn about timing; whether counter-postures are needed, how long interest can be sustained, etc. Out of their uniquely personal exploration, a teacher formulates questions for their students. Experimentation should be undertaken on one's own body before being tested on students.

Teaching should be the priority of all teachers. That this has to be stated is a reflection of the impact of the business model of yoga on the teaching profession. To strive or compete for more students may help the studio, but it is not teaching. The desire for accolades and increasing personal revenue is not teaching. Today, people often teach as a way of gaining status in the yoga "community" (it's not that they teach yoga … but that they are yoga teachers). When the teacher prioritises personal concerns over teaching, they have failed their students. Teaching involves honestly and freely offering information in a way that allows for clear communication and instruction. Teachers are inspirational because of the way they comport themselves, not because they aspire to be so. Teachers are both convincing and compelling when they have a method to express expertise on the subject they teach. Some teachers use their accomplishments in physical practice to express authority, but this is only effective if they can translate their personal practice skills into pedagogy. Ironically, a teacher is often best at teaching things they struggle with the most. This may be because they have had to deconstruct the posture or movement to learn it themselves.

Humour is a useful device and is effective when the comments are made by a competent teacher or practitioner, for the play only comes after mastery is demonstrated. Humour does not exclude seriousness. Serious or challenging ideas may be made more palatable through humour, and an exceedingly serious teacher may seem to be overcompensating. Humour is disarming and it may be used to make a point to students who challenge the teacher's authority. Humour may break tension in a particularly difficult lesson and show that the teacher is skilful and confident enough to be playful.

The Strategies for Sequencing

Sequencing is another skill set a teacher seeks to master. There are a number of options for sequencing that are not mutually exclusive and may be employed for different purposes in different situations. The choices one makes in structuring should not be gratuitous. Lack of confidence often leads teachers to copy sequences from others and, though there is value in looking elsewhere for ideas, these ideas should act as inspiration for the teacher in their creative process and not as a template for their own teaching. Novice teachers may erroneously believe that, if they mimic the work of others, they will, at some point, be magically able to construct their own unique classes; but this reliance will only stifle the abilities of the teacher if the mimicry acts as a crutch. Teachers may also want "clever" tricks and a large variety of postures in their sequences as opposed to keeping the topical focus small and exploring it deeply. Though variety may be seen as a way to sidestep boredom, deep exploration allows for a student to focus and better ensure learning will take place. Students are rarely bored in a class that draws them in and gives them a sense of accomplishment.

Many teachers utilise *set sequences* either in the context of orthodoxies, where they are already "optimised" for maximising the effect of yoga practice, or in open systems where they are utilised for various reasons. Set sequences allow for mastery and refinement because regular practitioners already know the sequence and can focus on the details of their experience. For example, Ashtanga Vinyasa Yoga proports a progression from healing to devotion in a number of set series, which are embedded between beginning and ending sequences; Bikram Yoga is designed for a progression from healing to ultimate fitness in two series; Sivananda postural practice is healthful "right exercise", which serves as an essential part of right living; Tripsichore Yoga has created set sequences with different levels of performance, which are progressive in difficulty.

Sequencing can also be structured around a *mini-vinyasa menu*, which allows for creativity within a structured philosophical framework – a menu of mini-sequences arranged by the teacher to provide a number of options for practice (e.g., Jivamukti Yoga and Shiva Rea's Prana Vinyasa). Mini-sequences may be classified by function or position in a larger set of sequencing rules.

Classes may also be sequenced to build to a *master posture*. A master posture may be a challenging pose or a culmination of a number of elements central to the teaching focus. The sequence of movements preceding the posture act as preparation. This highlights the relationship between the master posture and the postures and movements that precede it. This strategy encourages students to understand the progression toward goals. By focusing on small, achievable steps, the progression serves to expand the possibilities for students who might otherwise see a posture as "out of reach". All good classes have a component of this, but coherent progression is central to this sequencing strategy.

There are a number of other strategies for sequencing. One is to focus on *a point of learning* (these can be subtle or gross points, depending on the level of the class). Breath, alignment, body part, concentration, meditative quality, function (e.g., digestion, sleep, energising, grounding, *dosha*, and *kosha*) are examples of points of learning. *Repetition*, with or without variations, is another; it provides an opportunity for a fuller ritual experience. This breaks down barriers (fear, physical, or psychological resistance, complexity of execution) by repeatedly performing a posture (or related set of postures) in different contexts. Students are able to discover postures in a deeper way through a "layered experience". Finally, the *warm-up/cool-down* (exercise model) strategy provides an experience familiar to those in fitness culture.

In good sequencing, a teacher helps students cultivate awareness of and attunement to their internal state and the state of the world around them. This develops an appreciation of the constancy of change and the savouring of this inevitability. Sequencing should emphasise the importance of process, where *asanas* or *vinyasas* within sequences become tools for experience rather than goals in and of themselves.

INVESTING IN STUDENTS

Teachers should be clear about why the techniques they use fulfil the aims of teaching. Some may choose to couch these aims in anatomical or physiological ways and others in artistic or expressive terms, while others still put forth psychological or spiritual reasons. They are at their most convincing when they deliver a compelling rationale for how the student can feasibly attain what is deemed "good" through direct experience. After whatever talk, demonstration, or direct assistance is given, the student must find themselves closer to attaining this direct experience on their own. Yoga is not taught "to fix people". A good teacher encourages students to discover their own agency, through which they address relevant challenges in their practice and beyond. However, students will tend toward better outcomes from teachers whom they wish to please; these are the teachers that they believe "care" about them and their progression. If students believe that the teacher cares, they can be asked to take on more difficult challenges. Students feel an obligation to their teachers because their teachers have made an investment in them.

UNDERSTANDING COMMUNITY

A number of recent publications have considered the evolution of modern yoga and the reinterpretation of yogic aspirations in light of the knowledge gained through both modern science and decades of cross-cultural interpretation and experimentation. Sarah Strauss's *Positioning Yoga*, Andrea Jain's *Selling Yoga*, and Theodora Wildcroft's *Patterns of Authority and Practice Relationships in 'Post-Lineage Yoga'* explore the meaning of yoga for modern practitioners and provide what anthropologists identify as the *emic* perspective – the understanding of yoga from inside the community of practice. This term *community of practice* is interesting, for not only does it easily describe yoga practitioners from the language of modern yoga, but it also refers to an academic analysis of community and the way that knowledge is transferred. Coined by Jean Lave and Etienne Wenger (1991), a community of practice is a group of people who "share a concern or a passion for something they do and learn how to do it better as they interact regularly" (Wenger-Traynor 2015).[8] As Lave and Wenger noted, community of practice can evolve naturally out of the members' common interests or can be created deliberately with the goal of gaining knowledge. It may be situated in a place like a studio, but does not have to be co-located, in which case they form a "virtual community of practice", as is the case when envisioning the "global yoga community", or the "Iyengar community". In this way, we can understand

Wildcroft's evolution of post-lineage yoga; it is a community of practice formed around the desire to advance yoga beyond the disciplines of modern lineage constraints.[9] It is through concepts like these that one can understand the evolutionary potential of yogic philosophy and somatic practice, since, in communities of practice, practitioners share ideas and learn skills: ways of understanding and talking about yoga as a common interest. These communities transform and transmit knowledge and evolve unique ways of understanding their practices, sometimes independently of a formal teacher.

CHALLENGES OF COMMUNITY AND COMMODIFICATION

The challenge of "community" (virtual or otherwise) is that it is both freeing and an impediment. It is freeing because it is less tied to the dictates of a lineage (less direct oversight). It is an impediment because it is tied to the often unstated and unwieldy consensus of a group of individuals of unequal experience and ability in yoga. In this regard, it is subordinate to the local group/community and also the perceived ethics and ethos of larger virtual communities. The challenge for teachers comes when they find themselves at odds with either of these communities. Do they subordinate what they teach to the strictures of the larger consensus or find strategies to negotiate change?

As for commodification: what price the spirit? Does the ability to afford yoga classes lead to greater spiritual insight – especially if your spirit is not to be tied to materiality? Has such insight been presumed by the industry to be a luxury and marketed towards those who can experience the "aspirational good life"? What are the rewards that the industry promises – a deeper understanding of "self", a more meaningful and successful life, improved health and well-being, and heightened ethical discernment? Are these realistic aspirations for yoga teachers, practitioners, and studios, or as commodities, is yoga selling noble ideals they have no way to deliver reliably? It remains problematic as to how postural yoga, without a strong philosophic underpinning, might be fashioned to work on these things. Teachers are in a position of exemplars for most students and are charged with directing students as they work toward their goals. The teachers (with nascent personal practices) who parrot truisms about philosophy and its relevance to physical practice, do so because they lack the necessary experience and knowledge to articulate and communicate their own synthesis of the pursuit of ideals through physical yoga. If yoga is to deliver greater spiritual insight, endorsing teachers with the standards that are presently required for certification will have to be re-examined. The investment required by students will necessarily be of time and discipline, rather than simply financial means and aspirational desire.

The responsibility of the teacher is both awesome and daunting. Yoga teachers have the care of their students in their hands as they lead them through what must, in a good yoga class, be a challenging, sometimes frightening, and necessarily reality changing experience; an experience that may be characterised by frustrations and lapses in progress. Through this process students are vulnerable and impressionable. The responsibility of the teacher is to ensure that students are provided safe and honest instruction that is in their service. The manipulation of students for the teacher's gain – even when couched as beneficial – raises questions about what they are teaching. If students' interests are put beneath the interests of the teacher – be it financial, personal, or professional – it is not good teaching.

There is not a clear progression from student to practitioner to teacher, and so the choice to embark on the vocation through teacher training should be well considered. Taking teacher training should not be about learning the basics of yoga, connecting with community, embarking on a money-making scheme, gaining personal fame or esteem, or for any other reason than the passion for assisting students in their personal exploration. Prospective teachers should already be experienced practitioners who have taken responsibility for their own yogic study and who have already synthesised the teaching of their mentors in ways that are unique to that personal exploration. Loving yoga does not impart the skills one needs to teach. This ability is acquired (along with other skills) through dedicated study, self-reflection, and an understanding that teaching is not the same as doing. The adage that "those who cannot do, teach" is as disrespectful as it is false. For, to be a teacher, one has to go beyond doing – to a knowing that only comes through deep experience and thoughtful devotion to one's discipline.

Notes

1   Hindu American Foundation is a non-profit organisation in the United States that advocates for what they "believe is rooted in Hindu Dharma, and serves the

well-being of Hindus and the greater good of all." They have been vocal about the lack of authenticity of globalised yoga and see practitioners outside of the Hindu faith as both inauthentic and appropriative of Hindu culture. (www.hinduamerican. org/about/). Accessed 20 April 2020.

2   International Association of Yoga Therapists (IAYT) and Society for Yoga Therapy and Research (SYTAR). These organisations took ownership of the term "yoga therapist" and disallowed Yoga Alliance members from advertising themselves as yoga therapists, even if members were actually part of their organisations. Therapists could only be advertised as such within the therapy organisations.

3   QAnon, Anti-Vaxxers, Anti-5G, etc.

4   The author encountered this attitude when trying to get approval for an interdisciplinary college course on yoga in the curriculum at her university. The course was not approved because evaluators deemed it a "gym class", which required waivers for participation, despite arguments and a syllabus submitted proving otherwise.

5   Many studies show a high correlation between eating disorders and yoga, especially in the Ashtanga community (see Cook-Cottone 2017; Domingues and Carmo 2019; and Herranz Valera, Acuña Ruiz, Romero Valdespino, et.al., 2014).

6   These beliefs include pro-social justice, anti-colonisation, anti-cultural appropriation, anti-sexual harassment and exploitation, veganism/vegetarianism. (All act as sub-cultural alignments).

7   The relatively easy to access degree of flexibility and strength meant that the physics of balance in hitherto unusual or gymnastic shapes could be done by those who did not previously consider these possible.

8   The most complete work on this subject is Etienne (1999).

9   Wildcroft defines "post-lineage yoga" as: "Post-lineage does not mean anti-lineage. It can be commercial or traditional, radical or neoliberal, but it is rarely strict or branded. It just shifts the authority for deciding good yoga practice away from the absolute power of previous masters, to small community groups of teachers. The term therefore might be of wider usefulness" (Wildcroft 2018b).

Appendix 4: Reflection and Experimentation

Teacher training has come to replace the kind of instruction that used to occur in classes or mentorship relationships; it is now where yoga education (not just learning how to be a teacher) commonly occurs. It is abundant, but of variable quality. The idea that anyone can be a yoga teacher and that training is neither arduous, nor ongoing, has created a difficulty for discriminating consumers. Aspiring yogis are forced to search for good teachers and trainings, without clear standards for discernment. Consider what goes into good teaching, and the realities of teaching yoga in the context of its popularisation. Do you have a deep understanding of the discipline of yoga and an ability to communicate this knowledge to students?

4.1 ARE YOU POTENTIALLY A TEACHER?

If *dharma* is defined as that which is most appropriate for you to do with your life, are you suited to being a yoga teacher (is it within your *dharma*)? What kind of self-knowledge is necessary to answer this question? Do you have an aptitude for dissecting and communicating your understanding of complex processes of body and mind? Are you comfortable critiquing students? Do you have an aptitude for seeing potential in others and helping them to develop this potential?

What would you look for in teacher training that would enhance your abilities and address your weaknesses: to work with a knowledgeable teacher; to have enough time to process and learn material efficiently; to have teaching opportunities while learning; to spend more time on pedagogical work than on basic yoga skills; to have an in-depth study of an orthodoxy or an eclectic overview of yoga traditions?

4.2 MAKING SACRIFICES

Dedication to teaching requires sacrifices, one of which is personal practice time. The ideas you have built your career upon or the yoga style you have always followed may need to be sacrificed as you develop both your personal and teaching practices. Trends and business concerns may pressure you to teach in a way that you do not necessarily find fulfilling.

How will you find the requisite time needed for dedicated self-practice if you choose to teach? Are you willing to abandon the comfort of your yoga style or the ideas of your own teachers? What are you willing to teach to gain popularity or financial success? Would you still teach yoga if there was not money involved?

4.3 DEVELOPING A ROUTINE

When it comes to practice, are you wanting to *get it done* or *wanting to do it*? The creation of the routine of practice is necessary for your personal progress and as a source for ideas to experiment with in teaching. Routine is the recognition that some things are never completed and have to be repeated over and over. Routine can be thought of as a dedication of time, but it may be more productive to think of it as the repeated application (practise) of skills. Here are some skills that might be applied in everyday situations.

You may use your observational skills anywhere – if you cook, chop the vegetables, or assemble the ingredients in the cookware with a directness of intention, focus, and execution. If you sit for extended periods of time at your job, treat the physical experience as a posture that aids the accomplishment of your work. Unobtrusively and without comment, observe the bodies of your family, friends, and colleagues. What is happening to their joints and muscles? You can study the bodies of strangers while watching television. A walk to the shops is an opportunity to practise *ujjayi* breathing and its relationship to movement as well as the precision of the action of the legs. All of these exercises are ways of routinely addressing the skills used in practice and teaching in addition to the time spent on your mat.

4.4 ATTUNEMENT

Attunement is the process of adapting to your audience. The setting where you teach will shape your presentation and material – each venue attracts a different clientele with different expectations. How would your teaching be influenced by the following contexts: yoga studio, gym, health club, church basement, outdoor space, ashram, community centre/library, hospital, prison, school, day care? Which environments would you avoid and why? What opportunities would each of these provide for attunement in your teaching?

4.5 TEXTS AND EXPERIENCE

What is the teaching value of textual material, be it scientific, poetic, or philosophic? Texts (ancient in particular) are assumed to carry great authority for the traditional yogi. How do you incorporate textual material in your teaching? How well must you know a text before you teach it? Do you have your own method of evaluating textual material, or do you rely on others' interpretations? How do textual information and knowledge gained from experience intertwine? How do you test textual propositions in your yoga practice and teaching?

References

Agnew, Robert and Timothy Brezina. "Strain theories." *The SAGE handbook of criminological theory*, edited by Eugene McLaughlin and Tim Newburn, 96–113. Los Angeles: Sage, 2010.

Bender, Courtney. *The new metaphysicals: spirituality and the American religious imagination*. Chicago: University of Chicago Press, 2010.

Cook-Cottone, Catherine. "Yoga communities and eating disorders: creating safe space for positive embodiment." *Journal of The International Association of Yoga Therapists* vol. 27 issue 1 (2017): 87–93.

Curtis, Lindsay. "Lesbian body positivity: a yoga expert shares her tips for staying healthy." *Go Mag*, 4 October, 2018. http://gomag.com/article/lesbian-body-positivity-a-yoga-expert-shares-her-tips-for-staying-healthy/. Accessed 22 August, 2020.

Dark, Kimberly. "Here's looking at you: yoga, fat & fitness." *Decolonizing Yoga*, 6 March, 2014. https://decolonizingyoga.com/heres-looking-at-you-yoga-fat-fitness/. Accessed 22 August, 2020.

Domingues, R.B. and C. Carmo. "Disordered eating behaviours and correlates in yoga practitioners: a systematic review." *Eat Weight Disord* 24, 1015–1024 (2019). https://doi.org/10.1007/s40519-019-00692-x. Accessed 2 January, 2021.

Fouce, Paula, Director. *Naked in Ashes*. 2005. Paradise Filmworks International.

Herranz Valera, J., P. Acuña Ruiz, B. Romero Valdespino, et al. "Prevalence of orthorexia nervosa among ashtanga yoga practitioners: a pilot study." *Eat Weight Disord* 19, (2014): 469–472. https://doi.org/10.1007/s40519-014-0131-6 Accessed 2 January, 2021.

Jain, Andrea R. *Selling yoga: from counterculture to pop culture*. Oxford: Oxford University Press, 2015.

Khoshaba, Deborah. "Take a stand for yoga today: yoga's positive benefits for mental health and well-being", *Psychology Today* (online), 2013. www. psychologytoday.com/us/blog/get-hardy/201305/take-stand-yogatoday#:~:text =Yoga%20and%20Mental%20Health,and%20centers%20the%20nervous %20system. Accessed 20 August, 2020.

Lave, Jean and Etienne Wenger. *Situated learning: legitimate peripheral participation*. Cambridge: Cambridge University Press, 1991.

Lawson, Jill. "Yoga in America: where bowing to god is not religious." *Huffington Post*, 8 November, 2013. www.huffpost.com/entry/yoga-and-religion_b_4230240. Accessed 22 August, 2020.

Strauss, Sarah. *Positioning yoga*. London: Routledge, 2004.

University of Sydney. "Yoga more risky for causing musculoskeletal pain than you might think: injury rate up to 10 times higher than previously reported." *ScienceDaily*, 27 June, 2017. Accessed 20 August 2020. www.sciencedaily.com/releases/2017/06/170627105433.htm.

Wayne, Luke. "Hinduism and morality." *CARM*, 9 March, 2017. Accessed 19 June, 2021. https://carm.org/hinduism/hinduism-and-morality/.

Wenger, Etienne. *Communities of practice*. Cambridge: Cambridge University Press, 1999.

Wenger-Trayner, Etienne and Beverly. *A brief introduction to communities of practice*. 15 April, 2015. Accessed 16 August, 2020. https://wenger-trayner.com/wp-content/ uploads/ 2015/04/07-Brief-introduction-to-communities-of-practice.pdf.

Wildcroft, Theodora. "Patterns of authority and practice relationships in post-lineage yoga" PhD thesis, London: The Open University, 2018a.

Wildcroft, Theodora. "Post-lineage yoga." Blog post yoga and thought from Theo Wildcroft, 20 April, 2018b. Accessed 19 June, 2021. www.wildyoga.co.uk/ 2018/ 04/post-lineage-yoga/.

Yoga Alliance website. "Our standards." Lasted updated 16 December, 2020. Accessed 22 December, 2020. www.yogaalliance.org/Our_Standards.

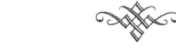

CHAPTER FIVE
THE EFFECTIVE YOGA TEACHER
FINDING YOUR VOICE

YOUR TEACHING VOICE

The discussion of one's voice will start with a clarification of terms; what is meant by persona, speech, and voice? One's *persona* is the expression of the character formed from parts of oneself. It is a presentation of self that is context specific and can vary. *Speech* is what gets spoken. What is meant by *voice*? It has multiple vernacular meanings; the sound of one's speech, the vehicle through which our words are spoken, and our cries and songs are expressed. But it is also used to mean the unique perspective of a group or individual, such as "women's voices" or the voice of an author. To vent one's voice implies the power to express oneself that was previously denied. In this chapter, "voice" will be used broadly as the expression of a teacher's perspectives, which covers a range of both physical and oral presentation. A voice may be unrefined and need to be clarified through the process of discovery. This voice is then crafted to express one's persona. There are many things that are out of the teacher's control, but what they present and how they choose to present it is their responsibility. The meta-message will be interpreted through the various aspects of the teacher's presentation; therefore, they manage and maintain an authentic voice and are cognisant of its impact.

THE PERSONAL AND PUBLIC

Teachers create a persona based on aspects of themselves that they believe are appropriate for their teaching; this presentation is created, yet separate, from their personal life. Maintaining a private self is crucial for the clarity of roles and the maintenance of boundaries (see Chapter 6). In turn, this clarity helps to ensure proper communication. Identity contains a number of pieces of personal information: sexuality, marital status, physical ailments, ethnicity, religious beliefs, etc. To what degree are these relevant to one's teaching persona, or, in contrast, what are the benefits of being a teacher who appears to be a more "neutral instrument"? Honesty does not necessitate telling people everything about oneself. Leading with an identity marker, even if it is apparent (e.g., gender), may unintentionally alienate students unless that identity is important to one's teaching (e.g., pre-natal yoga). Identity presentations may limit the way that the teacher is perceived and be seen as privileging one segment of the group. Likewise, the teacher's personal relationships may appear to privilege certain individuals over others. It is usually best to leave personal relationships, however mundane, outside of teaching contexts. One obvious example is the pursuit of flirtations with students, as it is both an infringement on boundaries and an inappropriately intimate portrayal of persona.

Personal stories of struggle and redemption may be useful when relating to students' hardships, but are they an appropriate means for teachers and what are the consequences of telling these stories? One has to honestly consider the intention behind sharing personal stories – are they about anything other than teaching? (Teachers may seek to acquire esteem, claim an unproven efficacy of practice, or even garner sympathy, rather than simply educate). Personal stories do have positive uses – they may serve to set a theme for class, illustrate a teaching point, or even create levity – enhancing the teaching rather than being the focal point.

Within the studio, there is no need for a teacher to reveal their status outside of yoga, unless it is relevant to instruction. A Doctor of Philosophy, though well-deserved, is not a necessary credential to be advertised to a yoga class, although, it will, along with other notable aspects of one's experience, inform one's "voice". To extoll credentials may be a reflection of one's need for esteem or validation, rather than an essentially noted aspect of persona. The teacher who asserts social credentials – "cool" – as a way of communicating their status rather than through the quality of the information they teach, risks being revealed as inauthentic. Dreadlocks, tattoos, mala beads, and symbolic jewellery have all become part of the stereotypic garb of a yoga teacher, but this display may conceal more complex dimensions of one's persona that are more useful for teaching. A teacher should be careful to select appropriate information to reveal (and conceal) and not fall prey to the pressures to enact a caricature of "yoga teacher".[1]

How much of one's ethical beliefs should feature in teaching? This is a question that each teacher will have to answer for themselves. If a teacher is a vegan, and strongly believes in the ethical implications of veganism, should they incorporate these teachings into their yoga classes, and if so, how should this be delivered? With an awareness of cultural sensitivity, how much right does one have to prescribe dearly held cultural practices (like foodways) into class instruction? These are complex questions that require introspection, and, if delivered, should be done with the understanding that ethical truths are relative, and ethical practices nuanced.

Teachers of physical yoga work with bodies that come in all shapes, sizes, textures, and colours, and have different ways of moving. They have smells, distinct markings, and they can be altered in various ways that are culturally preferred or prescribed. But, in the end, they are just bodies and are to be regarded equally. Though a teacher may have a reaction to a body that makes them uncomfortable (e.g., attraction, repulsion, or confusion), this discomposure should be addressed before approaching a student with instruction or corrections. Teachers should be respectful of the bodies they instruct, while acknowledging their potential for transformation. When a rock climber approaches a mountain, they may experience a sense of fear and awe, yet, if they are to ascend, they must focus on each hold and not be distracted by what they cannot know – the entirety of the landscape. A teacher approaches the bodies of their students addressing only what they need to enable assisting or adjusting. They are careful to maintain the privacy of both themselves and the body with which they engage.

SELF-STUDY AND PERSONAL PRACTICE

Self-study is the introspection and reflection that contribute to the crafting of a teaching persona; it is not a task, but an ongoing process. *Introspection* may occur while one is acting; *reflection,* however, is a process of retrospection. One articulates and speculates with their thoughts; they rehearse versions of themselves. Later, they may share these projections with intimates and peers as a way of testing ideas. If one cannot plausibly share these thoughts in comparatively safe circumstances, they will be even more problematic when placed before students. A teacher's ability to relate to students is developed both through experience and this process of intellectual discrimination.

Teachers seek to have a vast range of yoga engendered experience so that they can empathise with their students and their struggles. Empathy is an emotional understanding based on personal experience; it is difficult to acquire otherwise. In comparison, through mere familiarity and conjecture, *sympathy* may allow the teacher to "imagine" what the experience of students is like; but, when a teacher has *empathy*, they "feel" that experience – they know what it takes for a student to overcome a challenge and the consequences of this struggle. *Compassion* results from the ability to empathise; it requires doing what is necessary, even if it is uncomfortable or appears heartless to others. Feeling sorry for someone is not the same as compassion, and, as a teacher, expressing pity is fruitless. Being compassionate requires the courage to express what may seem like harsh truths. A teacher has the right to give a student information they believe will facilitate their learning, if they have overcome the same obstacles themselves – even if this information is difficult to hear. It is also just as important to understand the feelings of elation gained through triumph or the feelings of equanimity that come through mastery of the highs and lows of struggle in a challenging practice. Teachers must "know" what it is like to be a student. A teacher's past experiences certainly contribute to the development of empathy, but the *feeling* of these experiences may be forgotten if a challenging and reflective personal practice is not maintained. The need to challenge oneself – testing one's limits, questioning one's beliefs, and going to places that may be uncomfortable or unknown is essential. It reminds the teacher that this is what they ask of their students. Therefore, compassionate teachers spend time doing things that humble themselves and assess the feelings that these experiences bring. Though the role of the teacher is to be compassionate and caring, this should not be confused with the kind of guidance a parent gives a child. Broadly, a teacher gives information and tests the student; a parent gives love and affirmation. It is the role of the teacher to ensure that the student is well grounded in knowledge. It is the role of a parent to nurture. While their concerns are not mutually exclusive, the relationship between teacher and student is based on respect, rather than familial bonds.

Through practice, a teacher can distil complex experiences into their essential components as well as understand the relationship of these components to the whole. This dialectic process of distillation and synthesis creates a greater understanding of whatever material one seeks to teach as well as how to teach it. A teacher's skills should be broad enough that they allow flexibility of instruction. When one's voice is too restrained by self-imposed duty to a mentor or to an orthodoxy or lineage, this flexibility may be lost, and the teacher will fail to construct a unique persona with a distinctive voice. In such circumstances, the teacher is reduced to a voice for these entities (lineage or mentor), rather than a vehicle for carrying forward a body of knowledge with their own interpretation. The risk is that one's voice becomes a series of empty aphorisms; precepts that are nostalgic rather than innovative and that fail to honour their contemporary relevance.

Teachers also make sense of their practice experiences through discrimination. They evaluate their practice as a sensual experience and compare and contrast these evaluations as they vary from day to day. They learn to be adept at observation of themselves, so as to discover the range of their performance and how it relates to their teaching persona. A teacher can pretend that they are controlling all the aspects of their persona, but, through this process of discrimination, they come to understand that, once one enters into the experience of teaching, it essentially becomes an improvisation. This improvisation occurs within the structure of the persona and the persona becomes a vehicle through which self-knowledge is expressed.

Messaging: The Teacher and the Community

It is a good and creative thing to have flexibility in the way one presents oneself; personality is not fixed or codified so much as it is a process of identity making. Teachers are tasked with constructing a persona that is knowledgeable, competent, and compelling – a persona that is reflective of their strengths and interests; a version of themselves best suited to conveying the information they desire to teach. The persona that one constructs is important for developing both a teaching style and for cultivating a group of students whose interests in yoga are shared. A teacher adapts their persona to their students, to the content they present, and to the context or situation in which they are instructing. This facilitates communication and the learning process.

Yet, this adaptability of the persona may lead to a lack of authenticity if not honestly or reflectively presented. The authenticity of the persona is separate from the content of speech, for if a persona is deemed trustworthy, their speech is given credence even if it belies common sense. The tradition of following false *gurus* is well known within the yoga community. So strong is the desire to follow charismatic "authentic" teachers that the revelation of their manipulations is often insufficient to dissuade their followers.[2] Courtney Bender (2010), in her study of a variety of "metaphysicals," notes that strong beliefs in invisible and manipulable entities like *energy* and *intuition* predispose practitioners to other types of magical thinking that support the suspension of logical and demonstrable assessment.

The proof of indemonstrable "energies" lies outside of scientific evaluation. The yoga community, in promoting fringe beliefs and questioning established science, may more easily entertain or actively support conspiracy theories that reject scientific evidence. There is, for example, a correlation between yoga practitioners' beliefs and the theories espoused by QAnon (WNYC 2020). The promotion of these baseless theories within the yoga world had become so pronounced, influential teachers like Sean Corne and Hala Khouri (in 2020) made a public appeal to their followers: "QAnon is taking advantage of our conscious community with videos and social media steeped with bizarre theories, mind control, and misinformation – don't be swayed by these messages!" They continued: "QAnon does NOT represent the true values of the wellness community" (Wang 2020). Corne and Khouri's need to emphatically dissociate the yoga community from the messaging of QAnon highlights the impressionability of those who come to yoga, especially those seeking solace and healing. Suffice to say, there is danger in the power of the persona, where manipulative individuals may take advantage of students' vulnerability and pliancy.[3]

There are two potentially manipulative forces at play: the individual teacher and the community. The effectiveness of either force depends upon the student's primary sense of belonging. The message of the individual teacher is generally less powerful than the messaging established by the larger yoga community. As prominent members in the yoga world, Corne and Khouri recognise their potential to address a larger audience; however, despite a significant amount of media exposure, their power to persuade is not guaranteed. The effect of individual teachers' messaging is not wholly within their control, even for those who are influential.

The 2011 documentary *Kumaré* (Ghandi 2011) illustrates many of the ways in which the persona of the teacher of yoga is constructed and the dynamics with which students are drawn to and interact with this persona. Though from New Jersey, Ghandi assumes the persona of an authentic Indian *guru*, Kumaré, by manipulating powerful symbols shared within the yoga community. He grows his hair and his beard, dresses in a loin cloth and red robes, and takes on both the speech and the voice of an Indian *guru* with two disciples. His speech is reflective of well-known motifs in spiritual communities – it uses correspondence as grounds for interpretation (illusion = truth), speaks of the journey toward enlightenment through self-knowledge (the mirror), creates novel (and meaningless) yoga, meditation, and mantra practices (the blue light meditation), and promises personal empowerment ("the *guru* is in you"). Once connected to a yoga studio, Kumaré is successful, in part, because he exploits the community's self-fulfilling belief system; his message is consistent with their existing beliefs and expectations. He himself is surprised that he develops a dedicated group of disciples; even as he repeatedly tells them he is "a fake". These disciples are all seeking healing or relief from some variety of suffering, which makes them vulnerable and impressionable – the yoga studio owner who feels uninspired and inauthentic, the young couple in search of intimacy, the addict looking for absolution. Kumaré's persona is interpreted by his disciples through the stereotypic trappings of spirituality; so much so, that once he reveals himself to be Vikram Ghandi, months after his departure, most of his disciples continue to believe in his spiritual powers and maintain his identity as a true *guru*. Their desire to believe is more compelling than the truth of the situation. The disciples experienced a healing or transformation; an experience that they choose to explain through magical rather than conventional means. If Ghandi had been honest in his presentation, would his beliefs and teachings (the *guru* is in you) have been successful? How important is the means compared to the outcomes of our presentations?

BUILDING A CLIENTELE

Who Do You Want to Teach?

What is an honest presentation and what makes one believable to students? The persona a teacher enacts will determine the kind of students they will attract. A teacher who presents as a "coach" will attract those that want to be regimented and drilled. Teachers presenting themselves as discriminating and learned will attract students who desire the acquisition of knowledge. A teacher who presents themselves as a healer will attract students who seek healing or relief from suffering. To attract the appropriate students, the teacher crafts a suitable persona. To some extent, the student will see what they want to see in a teacher, if it appears to be represented in the persona.

There are three things to consider when deciding who one wishes to teach: what specifically interests the teacher, what is important to them, and why they are teaching in the first place. For example, a teacher may be interested in the phenomenon of embodiment, feel it is important to understand the intensity of experience it provides them, and come to teaching yoga because they believe it is a powerful tool for embodied experience. Identifying one's motivations does not preclude other beliefs about the value of practice or interests within yoga but clarifies the reasons for teaching and begins to delineate who one's student population might be. A teacher should have a profound passion for their work, regardless of the students they teach. There is sometimes a tendency to sneer at the idea of teaching beginners – as though this is somehow inferior to delivering information to those who are already knowledge-able. Teaching beginners is an opportunity to spark initial interest and excitement in the discipline of yoga. As such, it can provide the pleasure of watching students' progress and their horizons expand. In teaching beginners, one acquires the knowledge and skills to effectively distil complex information and present it in a more digestible form. Beginners may be easily frustrated or overwhelmed, therefore an effective persona should be understanding and encouraging and express the passion and excitement the teacher has in their own practice. In beginner classes, teachers present a broad perspective that offers possibilities for individual students and their emerging interests. It requires the teacher to renew their own familiarity with the subject and re-evaluate their theory and methods to ensure that they are credible and effective for the novice. One's first teacher is often their most important and influential; a student's progress in yoga will be informed by this important relationship. Teaching advanced students poses other challenges, as they may have habits that need to be undone, or they may resist attempts to alter techniques or ideas they hold, especially if these were hard won. Their previous accomplishments must be acknowledged, and unique interests encouraged in the process of further study. Advanced students seek the same thrill as the novice – increasingly profound experiences. The challenge for them is to continue to find new territory for exploration, especially if they are deeply invested in particular techniques or practices. Advanced students want to study with someone they believe is a more knowledgeable and expert practitioner.

The motivation for teaching may arise from other interests. To teach marginalised populations requires an understanding of the challenges those students face – whether they are based on physical limitations, social or economic inequality, age, or other factors that may limit (or be perceived to limit) access – and have the skills to adapt classes, to create an accepting and accessible learning environment. The performance of yoga will be an expression of the unique population. The yoga practiced at a nursing home will appear to be different from that in a prison, but bringing one's palms together at the centre of the chest has meaningful impact no matter the context or execution. Marginalised populations need to believe that the teacher understands them and the challenges they face in practice.

The efficacy of therapeutics is likewise premised on students' (patients') belief that they are in the hands of someone who is medically knowledgeable. If a teacher is passionate about therapeutics and sees yoga as a tool for healing, they will attract students who believe in a teaching persona that aligns with the healthcare profession. Though the physicality of yoga is arguably beneficial for the body, the attitudinal and affective changes created through an embodied practice (one that incorporates attention to novel ways of moving and breathing) have been shown to be significant (Virtbauer 2016, 1–14). In many studies, a greater sense of embodiment and a sense of responsibility towards the teacher (a desire to please the teacher or to have the teacher be successful), have been shown to increase a patient's sense of agency and lead to more positive outcomes, whether they be in treating chronic illness or relieving chronic mental distress (Loizzo 2018, 134).

Cultivating and Keeping a Clientele

One challenge for new teachers is the establishment of a clientele. This is difficult if one enters a studio setting where there are already well-established teachers as students may resist trying someone new. "Subbing" for popular teachers is a way to introduce oneself and one's teaching to new clientele. It is useful to know the original teacher's work so it can be built upon as one introduces their own material. It takes time to build a clientele. In small classes, one's presentation is as passionate as it is in well attended classes, and students should never be made to feel burdensome. Offering free classes to select students is a way to introduce your teaching and some studios encourage this, especially if it attracts students who are new to the venue, or if the teacher is remunerated per (paying) student. New teachers cannot rely on the marketing of the studio. They need to actively advertise themselves and their classes to potential students who might be new to yoga or their variety of practice. Selling oneself can be difficult to do but is appropriate when one has confidence in the integrity of their teaching. It is a measure of professionalism that teachers recognise the necessity to continually seek out new students and cultivate a clientele through the sustained and renewed visibility of their marketing. Ultimately, one's reputation as a teacher is the most important way to attract new students. Word of mouth is a powerful form of advertising, which emphasises the importance of maintaining a consistently high standard of teaching.

Experienced teachers extend their influence by recommending that their students take the classes of others. This expresses their generosity and self-confidence as well as the value they place on experimentation. These are attractive traits, and the lack of self-interest generates trust. It is professionally inappropriate to speak ill of another studio or class; in doing so, a teacher may be perceived as petty. Students will remain loyal to teachers for a variety of reasons. Chief amongst these is that they find the study of the practice engaging. Students may also be attracted to a teacher out of respect for their dedication to their own advancement as well as an alignment of their mutual interests. They trust the knowledge and skills that the teacher possesses. Students want their classes to be interesting and seek novel insights as motivation to continue their study, therefore a teacher works to freshly engage students through their own discoveries in personal practice and study.

TOOLS IN THE TEACHING TOOLBOX

Self-study may reveal skills that can be applied to teaching yoga. These skills come from a variety of experiences, within and outside of yoga practice. Knowledge of another somatic practice (e.g., dance, rock climbing, martial arts) will enrich one's teaching, as they allow the teacher to explore questions from different perspectives. This is also true with a teacher's other interests (e.g., painting, poetry, travel) and occupation (e.g., performing, education, law, counselling). Their teaching may be informed by these bodies of knowledge through the exploration of the connections between yoga practice and other theoretical concepts.

Interest in music or athleticism can serve as examples. Music has the potential to enhance states of consciousness. If the purpose of a class is "enjoyment", for example, pop music may be a key component, but, if the focus is teaching, music should be an enhancement. As with any aspect of class structure, music can be used gratuitously – it may distract students or teachers from practice (the playlist becomes the focus rather than the instruction). Stamina and athleticism may be a concern for a competitive athlete, and they may teach in a way that encourages these. As a martial artist, a teacher may compare the absolute focus needed in "battle" to the intensity they desire from their students. The dancer may choose to emphasise the lyricism of movement between postures.

Relationships with peers and mentors are important sources for information. New ideas are best tested with another set of eyes and ears – those whose knowledge and discernment one trusts. Mentors are particularly influential and valuable, especially for novice teachers. The information gathered from mentors is interpreted by the teacher and given in their own unique voice. The tendency to mimic is natural but fails to establish a convincing persona distinct from the mentor. Teaching is like a good cover-song, it is a tribute to one's teachers and mentors as well as to the acquired knowledge of one's discipline. One reviews and processes information before it is implemented; the teacher is inspired, rather than derivative.

The ability to demonstrate is obviously a powerful tool. When teaching beginners (to whom the postures are unfamiliar), demonstration offers clarity. When teaching advanced postures, the possibility of performing something difficult or frightening is better received by students when the teacher can demonstrate it themselves. When a teacher cannot demonstrate, they rely on their knowledge and ability to describe a posture instead. Detailed instruction assures students that the teacher knows how a posture can be accomplished, even if they are unable to demonstrate. This knowledge extends beyond the shape of a posture. It involves explaining how the breath is used, the energetic movement, the emotional context, the potential hazards, etc. A teacher's explanation may also utilise a student or assistant who can demonstrate. In any case, teaching requires more than the identification of a posture (either by name or with a photograph), it is accomplished through the evocative description of how a posture is performed.

TEACHING AND ETIQUETTE: THE RULES OF THE STUDIO

There are a number of rules, some of etiquette and others of ethics, that are informally enforced in vocations reliant on a clientele. These rules, though widely accepted, are sometimes overlooked in training, and how they are followed or disregarded will have an impact on how one is viewed by others. The manner in which a teacher shows respect for these rules reflects on their reputation as professionals. Teachers should support the studio that they teach in; this is true even if the teacher offers classes at multiple studios. Teachers should seek to positively promote the studio while advancing their individual careers, since, without the studio space and all that goes into maintaining it, there is no place to teach. If one teaches at competing studios, those classes should not be advertised within a competitor's space without permission. One supports other teachers at a studio, and their events and offerings. One way that this support occurs is through subbing. Teachers should make every effort to sub for colleagues when they are asked and engage with their students in a way that both assists and honours that teacher. Using subbing as an opportunity to deliberately "steal" students is inappropriate and divisive. When teaching workshops or courses in another's space, one should be generous by acknowledging the high quality of the studio, its owner(s), and teachers, and express gratitude for the opportunity to teach. Ideally, rules are followed to show respect for the profession and are not treated as either burdensome or restrictive. The grace with which a teacher manages these competing interests is an expression of their persona.

Respect for the studio is also shown in the way that one comports oneself. Punctuality is essential, both in beginning and ending classes.

Lateness communicates a lack of respect for the studio and the students who have taken the time to come to learn. Likewise, teachers should wear appropriate clothing, practice good hygiene, and be prepared to teach. Teachers should keep proper boundaries with their students and colleagues (see Chapter 6 for a more complete discussion of boundaries). A lackadaisical attitude or unprofessional behaviour damages a teacher's reputation and that of yoga teachers in general.

Though students are free to take classes with teachers as they choose, the "ownership" of clients is (informally) rule governed. Clients whom a teacher first encounters at a studio are the "studio's clients." This means that a teacher is acting improperly if they negotiate with clients for fee-based services outside of the studio. For example, if a teacher offers to teach private students at their home for a lesser fee, they are ignoring the fact that the studio invested in that client and, but for these efforts, the teacher would not have the opportunity to make this offer.[4] Studio owners take on most of the responsibility for the safety and satisfaction of students. Although individual teachers may be liable for their actions, the studio owner has ultimate legal jeopardy. The studio owner is responsible for promoting the studio and its teachers. As independent contractors or employees, teachers are responsible for promoting themselves within this context. A studio owner gives teachers the opportunity to acquire new students, but it is up to the teacher to cultivate and keep them.

USING LANGUAGE CREATIVELY

In the study of yoga, there are many sources of information (the raw material for knowledge), and the teacher is only one. Good teachers are alike in many ways; most want their students to learn to savour the process of meaning making through the development of a profound curiosity. As students gather information (sensorially), they process it through their existing knowledge constructs (they interpret through what they already know). The accumulation of this knowledge is accomplished through each student's individual process of meaning making whether this is within their conscious awareness or not. Knowledge is not passed down directly from teacher to student but is digested by the student through practice (and other experiences). Teachers draw awareness to this process so that students consciously explore in their accumulation of knowledge. A student may want the teacher to "tell them what it means", but a teacher's role is to offer information – it is the student who learns and derives their own meaning.

The Use of Metaphors

A teacher's voice is shaped through their struggle with the physical process of learning and teaching what they have discovered. Their teaching is given a structure (a beginning, middle, and end in any lesson) expressed through their voice and delivered with a rhythm, patterning, or internal reasoning, which acts to tie these parts together. This structure may move from familiar to unfamiliar, gross to subtle, simple to complex, or be a metaphorical journey; participation in this constitutes an imaginative exercise for the student and encourages them to be active in the learning process. Metaphors are a powerful tool, for they allow students to understand a novel concept through something that they already know. Metaphors also may attach affect or emotion to a concept and give clarity to its performance. Creative language can steer this process in the direction of the teacher's desired goals for each student.

A teacher uses metaphor to describe things that are not fixed or absolutely certain. Metaphors are used to communicate knowledge that is indemonstrable – because it is variable, unique to a lived experience, or an internal or ephemerally felt sensation. It acknowledges that the experience the metaphor tries to convey is not something that can be accurately described with words. Metaphors are used to shed light on something inchoate by its comparison to something familiar or easily understood. Comparative metaphors bring similar attributes or correspondences to light. However, they also provide contrast – the thing the metaphor describes is seen in the context of what it is not. The relationship assumes that there is similarity, but not sameness. Through this process of distinction, the unique qualities of things and experience are brought towards understanding.

Through the use of metaphor, meaning is created between teacher and student. This created meaning occurs in a neutral space (the *Between Space*) and it is unique to both participants. Once created, this meaning constitutes knowledge that is both shared yet interpreted distinctly by each. The value of a metaphor is in its ability to make sense of otherwise intangible ideas or practices not yet experienced. The student's experimentation allows meaning to be created without detailed information about the subject to which that metaphor is applied.

The adept use of metaphor is what leads to making meaning because it is suggestive. When it is suggested that doing a High Arch is like standing on a mountaintop and looking at the sky, it does not say that it is the same as that experience, but that there is something similarly glorious that can be found in doing the posture with a comparable perspective. This engages the imaginative, emotional, and intellectual parts of a student in ways that stating, "In High Arch, the chest is elevated, and the eyes look upward" does not.

Metaphor, Descriptive Language, and Naming

Verbal instructions may be conceived as metaphor, description, or naming. *Metaphor* is open ended. Description (either simple or detailed) and naming are more particular – they assume that there is an agreed and specific meaning to instruction. For students, the participation in (and understanding of) a teacher's metaphors is fluid and inexact – it leads to the processes of speculation and exploration. *Description* is precise and fixed (e.g., the legs are in parallel; the toes pointing forward) – in technique, it assumes that certain particulars are agreed upon starting points that are adhered to for exploration (the study of self and reality) to begin. Description is particularly useful for providing indisputable and exact physical directions. It may be used to disassociate a posture/ movement from students' existing knowledge and thereby encourage exploration and novel meaning making. However, it may also be used to support a codified set of ideas; restricting novel experience, as when movements/postures are instructed through a set script. *Naming* (e.g., Triangle) is concise, yet more generalised, and is assumed to be codified (interpreted the same everywhere). Naming alone gives no insight into the unique quality of performance. "Codified" concepts (like the naming of postures) make the imperative of meaning making less obvious and inhibit exploration, as the teacher and their students presume they "know" what the posture is and how it is performed.

When teaching technique, descriptive language is more precise than naming, and encourages the student to enter the posture with fewer preconceptions (students associate Triangle Pose with their past experience of that posture but are more open to other expressions absent naming). Preconceptions hamper the process of creativity and exploration and are the enemy of novel experience. This is akin to the use of *turning* in poetry, a device that leads the reader, if they follow, step by step, into the unexpected, where connections are revealed with delight and surprise. It also allows the teacher to experiment with form;[5] "what if we square the hip all the way forward in Triangle, as if we are reaching the top hip up through the spine?" or "let's see if our breath can seamlessly float us into Handstand, as if we are weightless". The use of descriptive language emphasises the metaphor of the "journey" and encourages the student to be curious about each moment of movement, rather than "hitting the posture". The spaces between postures become as important as postures themselves. Even within the four walls of a studio, "calling the postures" (naming) for a class is not the same as "teaching" one, for it relies on the previous understanding of students while failing to challenge them to explore the unfamiliar. However, one of the strengths of naming is that it may act as a shorthand when additional information would be superfluous.

The names of postures do have metaphoric potential; Warrior Pose implies fierceness, Tree Pose stability and growth, Corpse Pose stillness and surrender. Each name supplies not only an analogy but suggests an affect for its performance. However, putting the body into a form also has the potential to create an affect. In this light, the use of Sanskrit names for postures is not a neutral exercise. If a teacher chooses to use Sanskrit names, they should do so knowing why. Sanskrit names may serve to "authenticate" a teacher's voice as they tie them to what is understood as an ancient and authentic tradition. But they may also obscure the learning process for students who do not speak Sanskrit; by using Sanskrit names, a teacher may miss an opportunity to evoke a more meaningful experience for students. In addition, neither Sanskrit names, or more common coinages, are used consistently between disciplines or studios, so reliance on naming postures may lead to misunderstanding. This is particularly true for teachers who choose to teach in more than one studio, or those who appear as guest teachers. The language a teacher uses in their instruction is a powerful and important part of establishing an effective voice and should not be taken for granted. Naming postures (either through coinage or according to tradition) has drawbacks. Like any system of categorisation, names are bound to a cultural group with their own set of distinct meanings; they fail to have consistency both in usage and the nuances of meaning, especially across time. Meaning in language may be understood as having two components – denotation (reference) and connotation (sense) – the first refers to the essential definition of the word and the second to the connotations with which it is imbued. Though the denotation may be consistent, the connotation is shared within the cultural group and is the more powerful basis for inter-pretation; to the extent that it may even obscure the essential meaning. This is especially the case when words are emotionally charged or hold particular importance within a group. The term *guruji*, for example, may stand for an intensely beloved and revered figure to one group, and be the source of abusive opportunism to another, depending on each group's shared experience; the essence of the word has not changed (its literal translation – "dear remover of darkness") but its connotations are opposed.

Tone, Volume, and Contours of Speech

It is necessary to be precise and articulate when describing movements in class and one must be loud enough to be heard. To do both these things, the teacher must be clear about what they want to communicate, for when they are unsure, the students are aware of the tonal shift in the quality of their voice. Rhythm, tone, volume, and contours of speech are important components of presentation and can provide structure to lessons. The natural rhythm of breathing or one's heartbeat can act as an effective method for vocal presentation, especially when teaching movement. The voice can be metered to enhance the pace of movement and breathing. A consistent rhythmic presentation also serves to place the teacher's voice in the background where information can be accessed by the student when they need it, allowing the student to be simul-taneously engaged in the process of self-observation. Sudden shifts in rhythm can be jarring and can disrupt a student's concentration, whereas a teacher can be speaking continuously and, if performed with consist-ency, the student will generally hear the information that is relevant to their discovery and filter out that which is irrelevant at that moment. In essence, much of the instruction becomes a kind of background music to which the student finds a general mood for their practice, but that does not require full attention. The same can be said for other paralinguistic aspects of communication – the greater the consistency of tone, volume, and contour of speech, the more it allows the student to be a participant in their learning. In addition, when a teacher needs to make a point, this is easily recognised by students through a break in vocal consistency.

Though often overlooked, paralinguistic features are as important (and sometimes more important) as vocabulary and grammar in relaying meaning.[6] When someone is sarcastic in their tone, for example, the intended meaning of their speech may be the opposite of what was actually said. The conventions for structuring spoken language (assembling sounds, words, and sentences grammatically) and for its use (paralinguistics) reveal the relationship between language and culture. When tone, volume, and the contours of speech are shared within a community of speakers, these features of communication become less marked (imbued with social meaning). When speech affectations are unfamiliar, unusual, or stylised, they have the potential to cause disruption until their meaning is made clear. Colloquial turns of phrase are one example of this, and they are particularly distracting when a teacher is not aware that they use them. A teacher may, in their vernacular, frequently use phatics[7] in their speech; "like, you know", "it's sorta kinda", "we're gonna…", or "…right?". While these may seem innocuous, where these speech phatic devices are uncommon, they are likely to move the students' focus away from *what* the teacher is saying, to *how* they are saying it, and may also create a lack of clarity. This can be said of marked affectations or accents as well, since they draw attention to the mode of delivery rather than the importance of the content. This is not to denigrate any form of speech, but only to acknowledge that, the more "unmarked" the voice, the more effective it is in teaching diverse populations. Like any good stage actor, one modulates their voice to best play the character they wish to convincingly portray. Alternately, students, once knowledgeable of a speech form, will learn to ignore its unusual structures, especially if the teacher indicates directly or through nuance that they are well aware of "how they sound". The teacher's self-awareness allows the students to then disregard the differences. ("Oh, okay, she knows she sounds like that!") Likewise, a teacher who is aware of their marked speech may choose to enhance it and, in doing so, invite students into their personal space. Enhancement may utilise a variety of paralinguistic devices: gesturing, volume, intonation, or characterisation. The strategy may range from underkill to a more or less subtle exaggeration of their speech or gestural differences. By highlighting their vernacular, teachers express solidarity with their students and diminish the status differences between them.[8]

THEMES

Many teachers choose to structure their classes around a theme (some studios require it). It is fairly common for teachers to do a "reading" in class that elucidates their theme. The selection of a reading symbolically aligns the teacher with that of the author and serves to further define a teacher's persona, be it poetic, playful, spiritual, or some other identity. The reading can be presented in the beginning or at the end of class and is reflective of the beliefs of the teacher. Reading at the beginning of the class can introduce a metaphor; once introduced it may be manipulated to reveal other subjects. The more evocative the reading, the more potential it has for impact, but, equally so, an obtuse reading may require the teacher to guide students through interpretation. A reading presented at the end of class might better assist students in their reflections on practice and encourage them to create their own interpretations. The most control for the teacher is gained when readings bookend the class; the beginning introduces an interpretive frame and then concludes with an emphasis on that interpretation. This bookending "closes the circle" of interpretation and can be accomplished with one's own words or the words of others. Good classes have the right amount of "clarity" and "mystery" and it is the skilful teacher that knows which cards should be "left down" to maintain interest in the process and which should be "shown".

One's teaching persona is an expression of what one esteems and a depiction of one's interests and experiences – an enactment of what one stands for in yoga. It is malleable, it adapts to the audience, and it incorporates quirks and imperfections. It may be humorous, curious, intellectual, sceptical, or sarcastic. Though there are aspects of one's character that are necessarily excluded, one's persona is pliant, and its breadth is what makes it authentic.

Notes

1   We are making a distinction between character and caricature. Character is multidimensional; many aspects of a persona are presented; a character is well-rounded and nuanced. The complexity of a character shows a greater and more plausible range of actions and emotional states than a caricature. Caricature selects and stylises a small number of features and is quickly interpreted because its characteristics are

stereotypical and lead to predictable actions. This lack of range or dimension can be channelled for humorous or satiric effect. The yoga teacher as a caricature has become a comedy staple. Commonly emphasised characteristics are an excessively soothing voice and sexuality.

2   See the documentary film, *Kumaré*, in which an Indian-American man from New Jersey poses successfully as a *guru* in Arizona, along with other fallen *gurus* who retain their disciples.

3   See *The Guru Papers* (Kramer and Alstad 1993) for a detailed discussion of the danger of "authoritarian power".

4   A teacher may ask the studio owner if they can teach this private class (requesting dispensation) or negotiate a "finder's fee" for private classes lasting a certain duration. However, failure to disclose an arrangement with a client (of that studio) is unethical.

5   The idea of playing with form is not one that is shared across disciplines. In some systems, form is "set" by the progenitor or subsequent bodies. The notion of sacred geometry is one way to describe this "concretisation" of form. In these systems, if experimentation is to occur, it must do so inside of these strictures.

6   Intonation, voice quality, loudness, contour of speech, rhythm, and nonverbal communication are all examples of paralinguistic features of language and can often be more important in relaying meaning.

7   Phatic language has a social purpose rather than being intended to give meaning. In general conversation, they are commonly used as an unconscious way to get feedback from others in a cultural setting.

8   The style of speech that is the most natural to a person and is usually a version of a local style of speech.

Appendix 5: Reflection and Experimentation

One of the most important components of a teacher's presentation is their "voice" and the persona it projects. Voice and persona determine the kinds of students you will attract, and the standards by which you will be measured. Developing an authentic voice that clearly communicates with students will help to make your teaching effective. In establishing your voice and persona, you should be aware of the impact it has on your students and the forces which lie behind your choices. These forces include the evolution of the business model of yoga, the popularity of yoga and its image in culture, and the way that you present the purpose of teaching and practice. With this in mind, critically consider your responses to the following exercises.

5.1 YAMAS AND NIYAMAS

What are the "codes of conduct" in the foundation of your instruction? Do these extend into your life (and should they)? When one considers *satya*, for example, "truthfulness" – are there occasions when you tell something less than the truth?

Make up your own list of *yamas* and *niyamas* that you realistically can achieve as a teacher (appropriateness, clarity, timeliness, punctuality, generosity, dedication, inquisitiveness, nonattachment to the results of your teaching, patience, fairness). The *a-* (as in *ahimsa*, nonharming) and the *ni-* in *niyama* (non, as in nonattachment) do not tell you what to do; they instead indicate that your actions should be "absent of some behaviour" without offering specific alternatives. What implication does this have on your certitude when teaching ethics or prescribing the "yogic lifestyle"?

5.2 CREATING EMPATHY FOR THE OPPOSITE

Empathy is the ability to "feel" what another person is feeling. It cannot be learned intellectually and is gained through embodied experience. The strengths and abilities of one person are the challenges of another. Varied capabilities are perplexing to those who don't share them and pose a challenge when teaching. People's experience is often quite different depending on age, body type, confidence, strength, and even culture. It is difficult for the very flexible to understand the problems of the very tight, and likewise for very tight people trying to understand the frustrations of the very flexible.

To develop empathy and understand how to work with others' limitations or injuries, or to discover ways to modify your material to make accommodations, experiment with these: Use a strap to bind an arm or keep one arm behind your back. Use only fingertips, forearms, or fists for support where you would usually use the whole palm. Strap a pillow around your stomach and notice how you need to change your movements. Wear really tight jeans or layers of pants during practice to see what tight hips feel like. Strap your shoulders like a shrug, so that your shoulder mobility is limited during practice.

Flexible people are more likely to go into positions where they are no longer in complete control of their bodies. For example, they do not feel when they are hyperextending; they have difficulty integrating their bodies in inversions (it is easier to balance a pencil on a single finger than a wet piece of spaghetti), and they tend to surrender to gravity rather than create a resistance to it. How would you create an exercise to enable the inflexible to understand what it is like to easily surpass the limit of their physical control? How do you convince the very flexible to work within the limits of their control?

5.3 CORRECTIONS: ASSISTING AND ADJUSTING

Physical corrections are a traditional part of somatic practices because they are a direct method of teaching. However, they are only as effective as the skilfulness of the teacher. How do you assess the effectiveness of your corrections (physical and verbal)? When might you use verbal corrections and when might you instead choose physical ones? What part does demonstration play in your teaching and corrections? Are you effective at getting students to do things on their own once you have made a correction?

5.4 YOU ARE WHAT YOU SPEAK

Choose a posture that you believe you "know" but cannot perform (or have difficulty performing) and create a detailed teaching description. Use this description to teach this posture to students. What skills are needed to teach things that you cannot reliably demonstrate? What language devices do you choose to describe internal sensations, coordination of breath and movement, and the other components of performance you see as essential for this posture? Think of metaphors you might use to describe the aspects that cannot be demonstrated or that facilitate a certain quality of performance. (Examples: Perform the posture like you are levitating, open your ribcage like an umbrella, or do it like you are absolutely "certain you are correct").

5.5 THE YOGA COMMUNITY

Who do you respect in the yoga community? What is the basis of this respect? Do you think there is value in cooperation with those that you respect; those that you don't? Is there a value in sharing teachers and students, collaborating for workshops and training, recommending each other's classes and events? Is this cooperation happening where you practice or teach? What stands in the way of this cooperation? What benefits would (increased) cooperation bring to the yoga "community"?

5.6 THE BUSINESS OF YOGA

The business model of yoga has led to a focus on making money rather than education. What are the implications of this focus? Are you willing to work another job to be a yoga teacher? How do you feel about studios selling questionable products or services to make money if that's what people want, or if it supports the survival of the studio? What are you willing to teach/do to make money?

5.7 THE PERSONAL IS POLITICAL

Yoga teachers often begin or frame their classes around stories of personal struggle and redemption. The stories that we tell are not neutral; they are used to create and solidify a teaching persona and communicate values and beliefs to our students. Write out the personal stories (*dharma* talks) that you have told and think about the biography you are presenting. Is it authentic? What messages are you sending to your students? Are there ancillary reasons you tell these stories (entertainment, theme building, education)?

Pick one of your stories – a story of personal redemption, an anecdote to illustrate human fallibility, an illustrative metaphor for focal point of practice, or a story to make you relatable. Identify people who you trust to "workshop" your stories and give you constructive feedback. Are your stories sufficiently divorced from a need for self-promotion and are they effective as a tool for teaching?

5.8 A WORLD IN A GRAIN OF SAND; ETERNITY IN AN HOUR

The universe is vast, therefore finite creatures like humans rely upon their skill in metaphor and extrapolation to infer what they can about its nature and extent. The body, equipped with its sensory tools, feeds our minds with information from which we deduce. With the technology of the microscope, we can see teeming worlds too small to be observed with the unaided eye; telescopes and space exploration have revealed wonders that are both intellectually and imaginatively stimulating. The old yogic saw of "mistaking a coil of rope for a snake" can be reinterpreted in a twenty-first-century manner – from very close it appears to be a vibrating field of energetic particles and from very far away it appears as a single dot. Things are as they appear to be, but they are also much more. Interpretation is based on the relative position of the observer and conditioned through previous experiences.

What happens when you focus on a dot on the ceiling as you practice Sun Salutes? Can you focus on the minutiae (e.g., big toe) of an aspect of your practice without losing the holistic experience? Or is that the point – to observe the same practice from different perspectives and to note different somatic experiences? How might this subjectivity lead to very different conclusions when individuals have shared the same experience or information? What is the teacher's role in guiding these conclusions?

5.9 THE QUEST FOR MEANING

INTRODUCTION TO POETRY, BY BILLY COLLINS

I ask them to take a poem
and hold it up to the light
like a color slide

or press an ear against its hive.

I say drop a mouse into a poem
and watch him probe his way out,

or walk inside the poem's room
and feel the walls for a light switch.

I want them to waterski
across the surface of a poem
waving at the author's name on the shore.

But all they want to do
is tie the poem to a chair with rope
and torture a confession out of it.

They begin beating it with a hose
to find out what it really means.

(Credit: Billy Collins, "Introduction to Poetry" from *The Apple That Astonished Paris.* Copyright © 1988, 1996 by Billy Collins. Reprinted with the permission of The Permissions Company, LLC on behalf of the University of Arkansas Press, uapress.com.)

The poet Billy Collins has this aspiration for his students – to be connoisseurs of the written word through embodied sensorial exploration. How does your experience with teaching or being a student reflect Collins' concerns and inform the way you might value the exploration of ideas? What roadblocks appear in the way of the quest for meaning?

References

Bender, Courtney. *The new metaphysicals: spirituality and the American religious imagination.* Chicago: University of Chicago Press, 2010.

Ghandi, Vikram, director. *Kumaré.* Kino Lorber, 2011.

Kramer, Joel, and Diana Alstad. The Guru Papers: masks of authoritarian power. Berkeley: Frog, Ltd., 1993.

Loizzo, Joseph J. "Can embodied contemplative practices accelerate resilience training and trauma recovery?" *Front. Hum. Neurosci.* vol. 12 (2018): 134. https://doi.org/10.3389/fnhum.2018.00134.

Virtbauer, Gerald. "Presencing process: embodiment and healing in the Buddhist practice of mindfulness of breathing." *Mental Health, Religion & Culture*, vol. 19 (2016): 1–14.

Wang, Esther. "Eat, pray, conspiracy: how the wellness world embraced QANON," *Jezebel* (23 September, 2020).

WNYC, "The rise of conspirituality," Podcast from *WNYC* radio. (25 September, 2020).

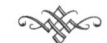

Chapter Six
Critical Social Issues for Yoga Teachers
Borders and Boundaries

> In considering criticism you have to make up your mind, first and foremost, what respect do you have for the person who criticises you. Do you feel from your observation and experience that they are worthy of your respect? How far do they understand the subject?
>
> (Gick 1997, 113)

THE ROLES OF TEACHER AND STUDENT

In essaying the roles of teacher or student, all might be seen as a form of play-acting or else a highly creative effort that each does in a uniquely expressive fashion. These "characterisations" give answers to the questions of "Who am I?", "What do I stand for?", "What is my purpose here?" and, of course, "What is yoga?" The solutions each student and teacher create to these significations of identity vary, and the appraisals of their auditors are equally diverse, but, ultimately, these characterisations must satisfy the integrity of the creators themselves.

The Individual and the Group

There is considerable pliancy in a well-formed character, but it must be plausibly based in the reality of who the teacher or student is in

DOI: 10.4324/9781003181910-7

other circumstances. Its primary purpose is to facilitate learning within the context of the yoga studio. One might ask, "Why don't they just be themselves?" Someone may be knowledgeable about yoga, yet feel uncomfortable about assuming the authority of a teacher. To be successful, they must overcome their "normal" social stance and brazen or muddle their way through this discomfort. Others revel in the attention or esteem they believe is conferred upon them. Some assume the models of teachers they have known – if they were stern taskmasters, they take on a similar demeanour, while others, for their own reasons, show resolve to demonstrate an opposing teaching style to what they have experienced. Regardless, there is no teaching style that pleases all students, but each portrayal functions to define and limit the roles and responsibilities of teacher and student.

Students intuitively assume their own kinds of role play. Some set their mats up front and centre and sit with erect spines as if to say "Look, I am the most alert and devotedly attentive student", while others retreat to a back corner as if to meld into the woodwork. Such strategies are an inevitable part of social interactions, but their influence is lessened by the fact that they occur in the context of a group. The central importance of the group in defining appropriate roles for individual students and teachers is too often overlooked. Klaus Nevrin (2008) argues that the practice environment itself is essential to understanding both the social interactions that take place there and the way that a somatic practice is successful in achieving emotional and possibly spiritual impact. He highlights Ben Malbon's (1999, 72–74) argument that:

> ...group activities will collectively involve a "collective sensibility" or "being togetherness" that can, temporarily at least, and given the right circumstances, unload the burden of individuality. Thus, by moving among and being in proximity to others, and identifying with others, in a group and with a collective focus...one can slip between consciousness and self-consciousness of being part of something larger, between anonymizing and individualizing. Moreover, sensations of belonging can be prolonged, as when one identifies with certain sites, times, memories, paraphernalia or others not physically present. These are forms of emotional involvement that seem to be quite common in [modern postural yoga] environments.
>
> (Nevrin 2008, 128)

Anthropologist Clifford Geertz has argued that "[n]ot only ideas, but emotions too, are cultural artifacts;" therefore, "feelings" (affects), are also cultural and no more individual or personal than beliefs.[1] Yoga practitioners often comment that they feel a sense of connection between themselves and others with whom they practice regularly, even if they have never spoken and without knowing their names. This sense of belonging is due, in part, to the creation of shared emotion formed in the studio and engendered through practice. Spirituality and emotional response may be understood as a "body felt sense" (Levin 1997, 180–181), a phenomenological experience that is "felt" in certain contexts and heightened when shared with others. Whether in church chanting prayers or in the studio performing breathing and moving in unison, specific emotions are generated by the group that serve to unify and articulate the shared beliefs and practices therein. The intensity of emotion a student may experience (as spirituality or ecstasy) is dependent upon their ability to integrate themselves fully into the group and master its evocative techniques in group practice. Regardless, the group enhances the intensity of the experience, as in any ritualised behaviour (see Chapter 2).

Nevrin (2008) also argues that this is not intended to deny the importance of individual experience, but that individual experience is made less ambiguous (and burdensome) through the influence of group expectations. Once a student joins a studio, they are able to choose a role that best defines them within this social context. No matter the status, this role is negotiated with others who occupy the space and is in line with the group's beliefs and behaviours. This affords the student an opportunity for the sharing of satisfactory emotional experience with the group and as an individual member of it. The comfort each individual has in their role is a measure of the assuredness they have as a member of the studio and this allows for students and teachers to relate to each other in ways that are appropriate to the conventions of the studio.

THE PLAY OF STATUS: DOMINANCE AND SUBMISSION

When the teacher engages the students, complex social interactions are displayed that demonstrate the relative dominance or submission of the participants. For instance, at the beginning of class, a teacher might be standing up, moving side to side, and occasionally gesturing while the students are seated; some sitting upright in formal yoga postures with their spines erect and their gaze focused on the teacher. Others loll on one hip while looking about the room, showing less attention toward the teacher. Though this is not open rebellion, it does imply that what is going on is not so important that it needs fully alert readiness. The teacher might pick up on these signals and begin to direct their words or demonstration with more vigour, perhaps targeting this to the "interested" students – emphasising and raising the status of one group and diminishing that of the others. Or they might feel that the signals of the "loll-ers" diminish their own status and they hurriedly get through what they are doing so they can begin something more stimulating – raising the "loll-ers" status.

The situation is weighted to help the teacher maintain authority. They may be on a raised platform; they can stand or walk about the room while the students are often seated and confined to the space of their mat; they can play a musical instrument (Tibetan bells, harmonium) or recorded music; they can talk at will while the students are expected to maintain prolonged silence. For some, this is a liberation from the constraints of their "normal" personality because there is in "real" life far more social negotiation – in the yoga studio, what the teacher dictates is the course pursued and strongly influences the behaviour of the students by projecting onto them who they are expected to portray. If the teacher (an authority) treats the class in a certain way, they will tend to behave accordingly. The student has less imperative to maintain an identity because being in a "group" absolves the need to do so – their social role is clarified by the way the teacher handles them and how the group as a whole behaves.

To present confidently to students is a performance that is relished by some and dreaded by others. It is easy to poke fun at some solutions used by yoga teachers – they have become a comic staple of popular entertainment as well as in the yoga community itself. The scatter-brained, misty-eyed, spiritually inclined *yogini* is as much a subject of humour as the exposed charlatan who espouses the spiritual while revelling in the material. Finding amusement in the sincerity of the dimly gullible or comedy in false piety can be found from Aristophanes through Moliere and up to the present day. Part of this humour is appreciation of how contrived these roles are. Yet, in "real life", we are forever contriving to give an acceptable appearance before others. People dress and behave differently for their bank manager than for their friends at the pub and are clear about what persona they wish to project in accordance with those settings. When faced with novel circumstances, the persona one assumes is still expected to be consistent with one's personality. However, to cope with the stresses of teaching a yoga class for the first time, some resort to stereotypic caricatures – a safety net to mask their apprehension. Though understandable, caricatures are unsustainable since they are two dimensional and are disingenuous. There is a difficulty as well with telling the shy or self-conscious teacher or student to "just be yourself". As long as one *is* aware of themselves, they are self-conscious and not responding as strongly to the external stimulus of others. Conditioned by parents, teachers, and social interaction, each learns that certain "honest" reactions are inappropriate – one displays "too much" emotion at the death of a pet or "too little" at the cultural travesty of inequalities and so disguises are constructed to make reactions acceptable.

The ways in which one expresses "personality" are subject to external circumstance, prevailing inner realities, and to the "props" one uses. Personality may be expressed through facial expression, body posture, verbal and nonverbal communication; performed in response to the reactions of others. Some of these manoeuvrings are under direct control and others evolve spontaneously. Students make choices that set a pre-disposition for how they will socially interact. Dressing up, one aspect of presentation, "is something in which most human beings take delight. One's appearance makes a statement about one's self – one's social status, one's taste, one's income. …People express themselves by what they wear" (Gick 1997, 120–121). When dressing up for the yoga studio, teachers and students seek to present themselves in ways that will make them successful in their respective roles and in accordance with their personalities. While dress and other aspects of comportment are creatively manipulated in the service of expressing identity, they are ultimately disposable or easily exchanged for other superficial symbols. In life and death situations, the trappings of personality do not matter; its ephemera, whether stiletto heels or cool insouciance, are easily shed. The "props" we use to identify ourselves are "accepted" by others, because everyone knows they act to ease interaction in social settings by providing clarity and structure, rather than being an essential part of personality. For example, if a student is thought to have suffered a serious injury in class, the teacher's role is to act in a manner that efficiently deals with the crisis and ensures both the safety of the injured student and the respect of the class, regardless of their chosen teaching persona. Eliminating the superfluous, while maintaining only the essential, affords the teacher the ability to act with a clarity of focus that is unimpeded by the trappings of their persona.

Self-Assurance and Self-Confidence

To feel appropriately attired for one's role in the studio may boost confidence, but, once one enters the fray, such preparations do not avail much, because there is a difference between self-assurance and confidence. A teacher can be confident of their knowledge, but still lack the self-assurance to compelling convey information to others. If one has been brought up to believe that it is unseemly for women to display superiority to men in knowledge or physical ability, this has an impact on the way information is conveyed or learning demonstrated. It may result in a female teacher apologetically giving critique or male students feeling frustrated and vulnerable when receiving it. These insecurities reveal themselves in wariness or obstructive behaviour – disruptions that are focused on social relations rather than the study of yoga.

Masks and Trance

Keith Johnstone suggests that faces become masks – that "[o]ur faces get 'fixed' with age as the muscles shorten, but even in very young people you can see that a decision has been taken to appear tough, or stupid, or defiant (Why should anyone wish to look stupid? Because then your teachers expect less of you)" (Johnstone 1979, 150). In a staple of mime, the performer assumes a mask that allows them to swagger mischievously, but tragedy begins when they discover they cannot remove the mask. They have become something they merely put on – something that is not the expression of their "true feelings". It poetically depicts the dangers of the roles we assume but ignores the pliancy we can employ. Strategies of deference or arrogance, humour or stern-faced seriousness, are assumed with the self-assurance of a lifetime of experience. These strategies work well for the individual, but they are not necessarily indicative of their confidence in the information they impart. Though a term like *mask* may seem too strong for the behaviour observed in yoga teachers and students, there are many areas where it is an apt description. A good mask – one that displays consistent behaviour on a variety of people who wear it – is noted in possession cults and theatre. The character of the mask is initiated and sustained by the permission of the group in which they perform – whether it be a voodoo rite, a Carnival parade, or a yoga studio. So deeply are we accustomed to the masks of personality that they may go unnoticed. There are archetypal characters found in the yoga world and their behaviours, which would often be unacceptable in the "real" world, are indulged in class. The braggadocio of the (usually male) maverick teacher strutting their tricks certainly bears comparison with the Capitano of Commedia dell'arte. This arrogance might appear comic to an external observer, but it is treated with seriousness by those within the class. The cavalier attitude a teacher presents through chronic lateness or the use of foul language is perceived as arrogant or offensive outside of the studio setting where it may, conversely, be admired as being "cool" or "rebellious".

The yoga class gives an occasion for things to happen that are masked in "normal" life. Every teacher, every student, and every class make a statement about yoga because they are part of the content of reality. This means that, regardless of how well we construct a teacher/student personality/role, we will sometimes betray that which is normally "forbidden". This may be as obvious as a flare of annoyance or as subtle as a lifted eyebrow. The spontaneity of dealing with physically difficult material exposes areas of emotional and mental vulnerability. But the content of the class does not lie in the personality and its conflicts with inner feeling – it lies in the yoga. Whatever the student (or the teacher) displays as the result of this struggle is "normal". Roles are emollients that ease participants in and out of the potentially stressful, yet deeply powerful, experiences. The postures, the sequences, and even the words used in yoga classes are ambiguous in their content – they are vehicles for these experiences. The teacher's role appears faked when they do not believe in the importance of the content of the experience itself. This confidence in a role comes from having been through such experiences.

Status Displays and Power

Desmond Morris theorises that "a status display is a demonstration of a level of dominance. In primitive conditions dominance is achieved by a show of brute force … In modern human societies … muscle power has given way to inherited power, manipulative power and creative power" (Morris 1977, 121). In the social displays of contemporary yoga, dominance is exhibited through physical prowess, as well as by displays of financial rank, the inherited association of "who one has studied with", and the actual skill one possesses through study. As flexibility is particularly prized, those who have it through anatomical inheritance are often awarded higher status. Revered or envied by those who are not flexible, this attributed status may be perceived as competition to the authority of the teacher. Strength and stamina acquired through diligent practice are also valourised and may be a source of status for students. Regular attendance at early morning classes where seasoned practitioners do "advanced" postures is celebrated, as is travel around the globe (especially to India) to study with renowned teachers. Innovators who have created novel styles of practice or are presented as iconic representations of the discipline are also revered. Authority and influence are attributed and negotiated within the yoga studio and in the yoga community in many ways.

TERRITORY AND PERSONAL SPACE

As territorial creatures in social units, the spatial interactions in which students and teachers engage may be understood as both tribal and personal. To give the tribe "direction", someone is accorded a dominant role and it is incumbent on them to "bring results" or suffer replacement. In a yoga class, the teacher is the designated leader and must fulfil this role by demonstration of their prowess or knowledge – all for the betterment of the class. Status is expressed through the control of space; establishing territory within the studio is both cooperative and competitive. Robert Sommer makes the distinction between personal space and territory:

> The concepts of 'personal space' can be distinguished from that of 'territory' in several ways. The most important difference is that personal space is carried around while territory is relatively stationary. The animal or man will usually mark the boundaries of his territory so that they are visible to others, but the boundaries of personal space are invisible. Personal space has the body as its center, while territory does not. Often the center of territory is the home of the animal or man.
>
> (Somer 1959, 247–260)

The first student into the studio might logically go furthest from the door so the room can fill up easily, but usually they will choose a place of personal preference. The next in must seek a place that suits them, but that if placed too far away from the first entrant might give offence and if too close might seem an encroachment. Their placement states, "I am dominant in my territory and you are in yours". Regular students, who believe they enjoy higher status within the studio, may assert ownership over a certain space, even if it is already occupied, or perhaps show disdain to the "intruder". In any space, people will seek to occupy a territory that secures their status, even if compromises must be made.

Territory: The Authority of the Mat

The mat has become an important feature of spatial definition. On the surface, it appears to be quite democratic in the way it delineates the equal importance of each student – the sizes are regular and the spacing between them tends to be uniform.[2] A variety of strategies are employed to clarify or emphasise the individual's importance. Yoga props, water bottles, clothing, and jewellery are arranged or cast around the mat, which expands the border and surface area of the individual's mat space. These personal items may enhance feelings of security and status – a statement of who the student is in the unstated pecking order of the class as well as a demonstration of their social ideals: "This is a metal, reuseable water bottle; not a plastic one". The extra layer of clothing they have on the floor could say anything from "I don't trust the teacher or the studio to keep me sufficiently warm" to "This is just an old sweatshirt because I don't wear expensive clothes to work out". Though one might be unaware of these choices, they are signals nonetheless and the placement of items is an indication not to encroach on this space. While the mat's use is primarily utilitarian, the brand or style marks status. An extra thick black mat has more cachet than a mat from a thrift store. If a studio also retails mats, students who buy them identify themselves as "regulars" rather than "interlopers".

The self-selected arrangement of mats in a studio is a striking testament to the cooperative behaviour of humankind – as long as there is the perception that enough space exists and has been equitably allotted, there is relatively little conflict. Informal rules exist to facilitate this – mats are arranged in rows with enough space between them so that body parts do not intrude into the space of others; and mats in rows should be regular in the direction they face. The way that mats are spatially arranged has an effect on the social dynamics of the class. Some classes are held with the mats arranged in a circle and some with rows facing each other. These present circumstances in which eye contact becomes problematic.

Prolonged eye contact is something that occurs in extreme intimacy or animosity. The look away from eye contact conveys either submission or dismissiveness and may be modified by polite smiles and small shrugs. When mats are arranged in rows, there is a tacit agreement that the front edge of the mat of those joining should be on the same line. However, in a crowded class, the mats need to be slightly staggered to avoid accidental touching. Though the logic of this should be as easily assumed as the front edge "rule", some see it as an infringement; "Why should I be the one who has to move?" The brisk authority of the teacher in deciding who must alter their position ameliorates this and is an example of how their dominance facilitates the social structure of the class.

Some people prefer to work without mats. In studios where this is not the norm, this can be seen as threatening – there are no obvious limits to that person's space, and they may be treated with perplexity or suspicion. "If they break that rule, what else might they do?" If the matless person distinguishes themselves with an exceptional yoga practice, others would have the incentive to try "matlessness". Were the teacher (the most dominant person in the room) to take up "matlessness", there would be further encouragement to do so. Desmond Morris states, "The higher his or her status in a group, the more readily he or she is copied by others" (Morris 1977, 19). Some may retain the use of the mat because they do not feel sufficiently worthy to try such "daring" alternatives. Other factors may come into play here – a person may sweat a lot and find they do not have sufficient traction without a mat. Similar situations occur when males remove their shirts to do practice – it may be seen as threatening if it is not the norm as it insinuates an infringement in a space shared by others.

Territory is an area of space that an animal defends as an exclusive preserve; a territorial species is one that "bear[s] an inherent drive to gain and defend an exclusive property" (Ardrey 1966, 1). Robert Ardrey observed that "man is a territorial species, and that the behaviour so widely observed in animal species is equally characteristic of our own" (Ardrey 1966, 1). He goes on to note that "possession of a territory lends enhanced energy to the proprietor ... the challenger [is] almost invariably defeated, the intruder expelled ... so marked is the inhibition on the intruder ... we may be permitted to wonder if there does not exist ... some universal recognition of territorial rights" (Ardrey 1966, 1). In the yoga studio, the notion that one's body is constrained by (and entitled to) a territory is so strong that some students will scramble about to ensure that their body parts do not get placed "off" the mat, even if it means they do something other than what the teacher has instructed.[3] The *territorial* space of the mat rarely needs active defence because, during practice, the exploration of the body's *personal* space has primacy. The mat accords each student their own "home patch"; a space that they alone dominate. Others are discouraged from transgressing upon this space and even the dominant teacher enters it provisionally. Stepping on to or falling upon another's mat is met with disapproval. Those who transgress may be the subject of gossip or other censure. Even the teacher shows circumspection about stepping into a student's space and will avoid it while making their way around the room. Although teachers enjoy dominant status, they must seek dispensation to enter the student's territory or to give them adjustments and assists in a manner that avoids violating their space. Teachers employ various techniques to avoid these violations such as crouching or lowering themselves in front of students, making eye contact as they approach, or seeking verbal permission. In this way, teachers are able to respect the boundaries defined by students while maintaining their dominance. Failure to do so may result in the perception of a violation of boundaries.

Personal Space

Personal space is a conception of the flexible way the self operates in a spatial domain – the space in which the self does not feel threatened – a home space. In situations such as standing on a mountain top or at the seashore, it can expand for miles, but while crammed in a subway car it might shrink to the size of the body. When personal space is diminished by incursions of others, accommodations must be made – gaze in the subway car, for instance, may shift to one's shoes or advertisements above the heads of the occupants. If it is so crowded that actual touching occurs, it is ignored or dismissed summarily with murmured apology. During yoga class, other students are similarly ignored – the focus is divided between one's own body within the demarcated territory of the mat and attention on the teacher. These actions are ritualised as they mark situations that present discomfort or even the potential violation of taboos. For instance, standing forward bends done in multiple rows present the possibility of displays of the buttocks while in close proximity to others. In such situations it is proper "ritual" behaviour to ignore this exposure by averting one's gaze. This disregard of transgression is signalled in what are termed "recognition rituals" (Goffman 1967, Hall 1973, et al.): where violations are left unacknowledged or otherwise given dispensation.

Transgressions that are unexpected and are not ameliorated through ritual action are potentially disruptive and may even challenge the status quo. Students who act inappropriately – enter exceptionally late, talk during class, ridicule others for their mistakes, undertake the role of teacher, fail to follow the teacher's instructions, wear revealing clothing, or violate the sanctity of the studio space – all potentially offend sensibilities or violate personal space, and these actions should be quickly addressed by the teacher if the magnitude of the offence requires authoritative action. This may be accomplished through humour or rebuke, in line with the teacher's persona, unless the offence requires more severe strictures. In situations of emotional volatility (e.g., crying, effusive laughter, or anger), the teacher manages the situation, not the other students. The emotional responses are contextualised by the teacher and the transgressive event may then become a potentially transformative or powerful experience; one that may be undermined if other students attempt to soften its impact through sympathy or co-identification. Such intimate experiences are interpreted in the personal space of student and onlookers alike.

Leading in the Dance of Status

Our aspirations, social ideals, and relationships are played out in an ever-shifting dance of eye movement, body postures, gestures, and verbalisations that occur in the territory at the boundaries and within the borders of others' personal space. In a yoga class, the leader of this dance is the teacher, and each student plays out their own variations within this construct. The teacher evaluates the actions of their students in this shared space and speculates on the students' intentions. A student listening to a teacher might shift their weight into one hip, lean backwards, look at the floor, cross their arms as if to form a barrier, and utter a sound like "hmm". This could mean that they disagree or are suspicious of what the teacher is saying, or that they are simply cold – or both – or neither. Yet, these are the cues that one uses to mould what comes next. The teacher might respond by leaning forward, turning their head toward the student, speaking more vehemently, and chopping with the hand – forcibly making their teaching point by moving their body and attention into that student's "space". Or, they might ask if the heat needs to be higher and humbly retreat toward the thermostat like the student's servant. Meaning is negotiated in social interactions and communicated in space through gesture and verbalisations. Playing low status can be as effective as playing high status within these negotiations, since a status presentation (demeanour) requires the appropriate social response (deference) (Goffman 2009). A teacher may intentionally lower their status by assuming a deferential posture and tone of voice, which will raise the student's status in comparison. When the teacher humbles themselves (lowering their status), the student is obliged to respond by acknowledging the generosity of the teacher. Doing otherwise will be perceived as anti-social and others in the group may censure them; also, the teacher may be justified in reasserting overt dominance. An adept teacher understands the dynamics of status play and shifts between high and low status as the circumstances demand to effectively maintain control; this is accomplished with the tacit approval of the students.

Much of a teacher's authority and students' place in the pecking order is expressed spatially. Those who have the greatest dominion of space rank higher. There is a *circle of deference* maintained by what may seem remarkably small and unconscious attributes. Someone standing with a deflated chest, a curved spine, and their arms slightly in front commands less space than a person with an elevated chest who holds their arms to the side and away from their body. Closing off the body with crossed arms limits one's spatial dominance – though it may make the doer feel more secure and protected – they will defend their patch; but are not in a position to acquire more territory.

The locking of eyes may be used by students to hold the teacher's attention. This forces the teacher to either reciprocate (implying intimacy) or to gaze elsewhere (floor or mid-distance) to show "listening". Though done from a position of low status, this disruption of normal back and forth implies or demands a greater intimacy and appears to raise the student's status vis-a-vis others in the room (creating possible resentment). The demand for attention from the teacher is an incursion into the teacher's circle of deference. There are innumerable ways status negotiations are played out between individuals within groups.

The degree to which the body is exposed can be another way in which status is contested in the practice setting. The teacher, because of their dominance, sets the standard for how, and the degree to which, the body is revealed or concealed. Clothing can be used as bodily adornment, but in yoga (as elsewhere) it also serves more practical functions – for mobility and appropriate coverage. Though some degree of modesty is usually required, there are occasions where students, either unfamiliar with studio attire, or those wanting to assert their dominance, will wear inappropriate clothing (or lack thereof). This can take many forms – students might wear revealing or ostentatious dress to call attention to themselves; they may wear clothing that is too loose-fitting or too transparent; or they may violate the sanctity of the studio by entering in shoes. Students may seek to gain status by mimicking the garb of the teacher – in costume or accessories (mala beads, sacred jewellery, or even more permanent modifications of the body like tattoos or piercings). The teacher may be given the privilege of exposing their bodies when others cannot, either for the practical purpose of instruction, or as a status display – one which highlights their relative physical perfection. If students in the class mimic this behaviour, they are conspicuously acting to raise their status. When the teacher is male and teaches without a shirt, this only affords men in class the similar opportunity to raise their status; conduct that may be resented by female students. It is the teacher's role to manage these areas of potential conflict so that focus remains on the practice of yoga and not on the inevitable dance of status.

The Student: Following the Lead

The role of the student is learned. While such roles vary between practice settings, there are commonalities. The student is of lower status than the teacher and acts in ways that express this to communicate respect and the acceptance of their role. The student has both agency and responsibility in accord with their status. The teacher's responsibility is to present information in a clear and accessible way, and it is the students' responsibility to learn. The student is also responsible to act with *critical acceptance* when it comes to the teacher's instructions and assume responsibility for their own practice. When the teacher instructs, for example, "If you can't do the breath, don't go further," the student must follow this advice rather than pushing themselves past what the teacher has clearly defined as their limit.

Students will sometimes challenge the authority of the teacher by asserting status. Because flexibility or strength or the ability to perform tricks may be valourised in the studio context, a student who is adept physically may incorrectly assume that superior physicality translates into knowledge (and status). Physically talented students may attempt to teach others during class or do things "their own way" in opposition to the instruction offered by the teacher; they may also disregard corrections or instructions offered to the group during class, or, instead, anticipate what is coming and move forward alone. Another way to challenge a teacher is by making "statements" posed as "questions". Through these, students state their own opinions: "I have always been told…" or alternately "Isn't it true that…?" or "But, I've always done it this way". Many questions are meant to raise the status level of the student rather than seek information – these may not be a deliberate attempt to undermine the authority of the teacher, but rather to seek validation through the display of their own knowledge or experience. In the context of a class, one student's genuine, yet incessant, questions can derail a teacher's message and other students may become frustrated. In such cases, the teacher must dispense with the obstructive student with immediacy. In private conversation, the teacher may take more time answering a student's numerous questions but is under no obligation to do so. Peers, who feel they are friends with an instructor outside of the studio setting, may try to assist them. Suffice to say, the teacher is the only one who should be instructing during class; all others who attempt to assist risk undermining the status relationships in the studio. It is unfortunate when there are teachers or aspiring teachers practicing in class who fail to give deference to the instructor. This kind of challenge is disrespectful and fails to model proper student behaviour.

Teachers are important models for demonstrating the role of "student". Some strategies for role modelling are risky because they potentially threaten the maintenance of the teacher's authority, but, if managed properly, can be effective. Teachers who practice with their students (and risk failure) in another teacher's class, encourage experimentation, perseverance, and humility. When a teacher is seen to fail while practising with an instructor of lesser or equal status, they risk a loss of status. When practising with a guest teacher who is an expert, a teacher models the way one shows respect for a higher status individual. Teachers who encourage students to explore other forms of practice, and present their own methods as provisional, highlight the necessity to engage in experimentation and discrimination and not to rely on any one teacher for affirmation or information. This empowers students to make healthy and intelligent choices. Students should not be encouraged to become teachers before they are adept practitioners; this confuses the distinction between the status and role of each. If "anyone can be a teacher", how is a student to understand the knowledge and authority that the teacher holds, and whether it is deserving of respect?

Dealing with these situations is a delicate dance of status, for everyone's participation should be validated. Teachers should act in ways that quickly diminish disruption, avoid an escalation of conflict, and allow students to continue with the business of learning. The idea of a democratically operational space is but a "shared fiction". The teacher is the only one in the room who is responsible and who is accountable for every student's safety and well-being.

Membership in the Tribe

Humans are social beings and will seek out social connections. Social groupings act on the macrolevel (e.g., industry and vocational organisations like Yoga Alliance, IYNA [Iyengar Yoga National. Association], and IAYT [International Association of Yoga Therapists]) and microlevel (e.g., the studio or *sangha*). The importance of *community* is so strongly endorsed in the yoga world that it is affectionately described as the *tribe*. Tribalism emphasises both the closeness of the relationships and its functional role. But, as with all kinds of political organisations (that is what a tribe is),[4] their primary role is to enforce social control and resolve conflicts when they arise. In other words, the tribe has authority and exerts dominance of one sort or another over the group. It is from the tribe that the teacher most likely is afforded their authority (through certifications, memberships, and other modes of validation) and from which it can be taken away. The identity of the tribe is beyond the individual teacher even if they are the progenitor (e.g., John Friend – Anusara Yoga, Amrit Desai – Kripalu Yoga, Bikram Choudhury – Bikram Yoga). The studio determines many of the rules that serve to organise and control behaviour – the temperature of the room, the positioning of the mats, the length of classes, proper attire, and the social etiquette – these are all agreed upon and enforced by the tribal members.

Tribes, because of their egalitarian ethic, have a tendency toward instability, internal divisions, and fluidity as they require a general consensus of the group. Their leaders are provisional, they gain or lose authority and influence based on their reputation within the group. In fact, the tribe does most of the policing of its members. The desire to belong allows the tribe to influence members to accept certain beliefs and behaviours through informal means rather than formal laws or strictures (Brown, McIlwraith, and Tubelle de González 2020, 152–160). This means that there is a constant and robust play for status based on displays and the fostering of internal alliances, which may not be as pronounced in organisations without tribal identity. When tribal identity is strong, it both fosters allegiance to the group and creates a dependence upon it. Tribes provide loyalty, support, care, and friendship to their members, which is often emotionally charged. The identity and status of the individual is validated by their membership in the tribe. When conflict arises within the tribe, negotiations fail, and consensus cannot be reached, tribes may fracture sending dissenting members to establish their own competing tribal entities.

It can be perplexing to join a studio when this membership is accompanied by a necessity to "belong" – to be a part of the tribe – as this allegiance does not have much to do with the actual practice of yoga. Petty disagreements or disappointments may feel like betrayals of trust or violations on a personal level because of the investment made in tribal identity and the accompanying emotional stakes. The dance of status, and the need to position oneself properly within the tribe, encourages students who have significantly invested in these relationships to remain in (what may later be defined as) abusive situations with teachers or other tribal members. When deeply invested, members may also feel as though they are "nothing" without the group, and this can foster continued dependence. This is at odds with the educational goals of creating students who develop beyond the teacher and who are independent of them. A teacher strives to facilitate an increase in status for their students through the acquisition of knowledge, and, if they are successful at this, they raise their own. Ideally, the roles of teacher and student regulate behaviour within the studio in a mutually beneficial way to facilitate the study of yoga, rather than play out a social drama.

VINYASA AND ASANA AS METAPHOR

There are many aspects of the studio setting that require and impose restraint; the borders of the mat, regulations about talking, the rules for comportment, the negotiation of appropriate status. But, in the arguably ancient performance of supplications to the forces of the natural and supernatural, as with Sun Salutations (*suryanamaskar*),[5] one can ritually extend past these borders and boundaries and experience a sense of "freedom" or liberation. The range of movements in *vinyasa* go from the extremes of expansiveness and grandeur to the most physically low forms of abasement, as one moves from a standing high arch through bowing into a forward bend and into prostration. One exposes and projects one-self into the grandeur of reality as well as humbling oneself before it. The truly relevant boundaries of this process are self-imposed. They are the boundaries imposed on the self by the self. These boundaries curtail the self's ability to understand the nature of reality, by the way they limit its definition. The boundary of the mat is such a restrictive territory. The mat is a feature of this self-imposed limitation and may psychologically limit the ambition of the student, since their intention is to abide by the strictures of the mat and its circumference.

Other self-ascribed boundaries restrict notions of the self through the labels of identity. Identity markers such as race, gender, age, social status, and disability all serve to limit one's potential – "I am not someone who does a handstand", "I am a visual learner", "I am too fat". These are artificial explanations; they are cultural constructions used to make sense of the diversity and complexity of the human experience. In an *asana* practice, through the approximation of stillness in the body and mind, one seeks to experience the essentiality of pure consciousness, the presumed changeless foundation of the universe – to see everything in the smallest thing. The *vinyasa* practice, on the other hand, invites the yogi to expand outward, to engage in discovery of an ever-changing limitless process. In a yoga class, where the mind is encouraged to explore its furthest reaches, people still impose unnecessary restrictions on themselves; "I can't do that – my body limits my mind and my mind limits my body" – rather than, "My mind can go beyond the restrictions of a reality apprehended by the senses".

THE MEANING AND IMPORTANCE OF TOUCH

Touch is one means by which human beings communicate. Touch has the ability to transmit a wealth of information and is never without meaning. Therefore, it is the teacher's responsibility to give touch that has specific and clear intent. Touch should never be gratuitous, nor should it be given for any purpose but to communicate clearly an instruction for practice. Caring touch and massaging are not aspects of teaching, but instead communicate a different kind of relationship between teacher and student, one that may be misinterpreted or blur the proper boundaries between them. Touch that lies outside of the communication of information about yoga practice is unnecessary and can be improper.

Touch is a basic human need that is essential for human development (Carissa, Cascio, Moore, and McGlone 2020). Touch can be understood as functioning within two different neurological subsystems: affective touch and discriminative touch. *Discriminative* touch is fairly straightforward as it simply sends information from receptors to the brain that define "what" is being felt, whereas *affective* touch requires interpretation of the meaning of another's touch; which may range from "orgasmically pleasant to excruciatingly unpleasant," and is further complicated by its "inextricable links to context, gender and sexuality, culture, and other individual, interpersonal, and societal factors" (Ellingsen, Leknes, Løseth, Wessberg, and Olausson 2016). Two main contextual factors are: 1) the partner in the exchange ("who" is delivering the touch), and 2) the intent behind the tactile stimulation ("why" it is being delivered). Touch is interpersonal; that is, it is shared between people who have some relationship to one another; whether it is intimate, a long-term relationship, or a more superficial one. Between intimate partners, affective touch is powerful. The greater the perceived intimacy of a relationship, the more that touch is imbued with meaning. Touch functions in many important and powerful ways; with touch, humans seek affection, express emotion, create social connection, communicate needs, express comfort or empathy, and establish and maintain social hierarchies. When one is touched, particular areas of the brain are activated, influencing thought processes, reactions, and physiological responses. Studies of brain scans have shown that affective touch activates the orbitofrontal cortex, a brain region associated with learning and decision-making as well as with emotional and social behaviours (Morrison, Löken, and Olausson 2010). In other words, touch can actually enhance the learning process. It is therefore natural that some students will come to class desiring touch. This may be especially so if that touch is lacking outside of the studio setting. Teachers should be aware of their students' and their own reasons for desiring or avoiding touch, and make sure that their own motivation for giving physical adjustments, like all other aspects of teaching, is clear, deliberate, and purposeful.

A teacher gains considerable information about a student through touch. They may be able to apprehend a student's mental and emotional state, and better understand a student's body – where it is unstable, how it moves, or whether there is unnecessary tension. What a teacher learns from a student through touch is both personal and private. It should not be shared with others; this information should be used only in the service of teaching yoga. Speculation about a student's emotional state does not qualify a yoga teacher to act as a therapist, nor should they want to blur healthy boundaries that clearly define the role of teacher and student. The resulting role confusion could potentially lead to misunderstanding between teacher and student. Teachers who are unaware of the importance of touch risk jeopardy when giving physical adjustments.

Improper touch generally occurs with good intentions. Some teachers feel the need to touch everyone in the room because they believe that it communicates caring to the student. This is a perfectly appropriate reason to adjust, as long as that caring is expressed through teaching. When a teacher corrects a student, and assists them in practice, it intrinsically expresses caring; no other form of touching is needed. Teachers must be aware that touch is not always welcome and not always appropriate. To reduce the chance of miscommunication, teachers can employ a number of "recognition rituals". They might crouch to get on the student's level, and, by reducing their status, make it easier for the student to accept or reject the teacher's touch. When approaching, they may use a softer tone of voice, offer a pre-emptive apology, or move toward the adjustment slowly. All of these strategies serve to reduce the threat imposed by the impending violation of personal space or allow the student opportunity to reject it altogether. When adjusting a student, teachers might avoid direct eye contact, turn their head so that they are not breathing on them, and avoid touching a student's body in any way that is unnecessary, steering clear of using their own breasts or genital area as the means for giving touch. Whether touch produces a positive or a negative effect is also dependent on the context in which it occurs. Touch will achieve the desired effect if it is performed in the context of teaching for the facilitation of student learning.

Touch is a sign of one's authority and the right to touch is the prerogative of the teacher. The teacher may extend this right to ask students to touch each other (partner work, mutual support). When a teacher confers the right to touch on students, they must be confident that this touch is both welcome and appropriate for everyone. There are those who do not wish to be touched by other students and may feel pressured to participate in these physical interactions. Sometimes students seek a teacher's attention; they may desire comfort, empathy, or connection with the teacher through touch. Despite a student's legitimate need for such comfort, the teacher is compelled to refrain from touch that is unnecessary for instruction. Gratuitous, ambiguous, or over-attentive touching may result in loss of the teacher's authority in the eyes of other students, and the potential for misunderstanding about the nature of the student/teacher relationship. The roles of student and teacher should be kept distinct and clearly defined.

SOMATIC DOMINANCE

The term *somatic dominance* has recently figured largely in discourse about yoga teaching – usually with pejorative connotations. In both overt and implied ways, it has come to mean something that is wrongly done by teachers who have inappropriately used their position to gain what is seen as a too intimate physical, emotional, imaginative, and/or intellectual dominance over their students. There are two key concepts – "somatic" and "dominance" – though it is true that one can abuse or take advantage of a student in a number of ways, *somatic* dominance relates to some form of control over the student's *body*. The teacher's body may be used as a vehicle to dominate. For example, a teacher might force someone into a physical position and injure them through this adjustment (physically or mentally), or likewise a teacher may berate someone about their physical skill and force them to injure themselves. However, modern postural yoga is a somatic practice, and therefore, inevitably, a teacher will dominate the student's body to some extent by virtue of their instruction. The elusiveness of what constitutes inappropriate or abusive dominance is problematic.[6] Therefore, the onus is on the teacher to create clarity and practise caution both when making corrections and when directing students' practice. If a teacher is working from a theory and method that make clear what the outcomes of practice should be, students are better able to evaluate the appropriateness of corrections made during instruction. The techniques that are used to enact proper movement or form (postures) support these outcomes and make clear why the instruction is being given. This clarity lessens the ambiguity that might allow inappropriate or abusive dominance to occur, or misunderstandings about the intention of corrections.

The teacher's authority is substantiated by their expertise in yoga and their ability to effectively transmit this knowledge through teaching. Observational, analytical, and communicative skills express this authority.

Experienced teachers have the foresight to develop goals and strategies that will accomplish this. They set standards and ambitious goals for themselves and their students that are also realistic and achievable. Their corrections are meant to bring those standards to fruition. In spite of this, teachers are not "perfected" individuals – they may display irritation, impatience, anger, indifference, or even attraction. When this occurs, a teacher acknowledges their lapse to re-establish the proper relationship so they can move on with instruction. If the expectation is that the teacher is to be "kind", "compassionate", and "non-judgemental", their corrections and critique may be seen as inappropriate or abusive, if they appear in conflict with the qualities of their persona.

In yoga, students are often placed in vulnerable positions. They may have their eyes closed; they may be lying on the ground in Corpse Pose (*savasana*); they might have vulnerable or private parts of their bodies "exposed" in class. When the teacher enters their personal space, the student has little defence. At times, they must submit to the touch/ presence of the teacher, who should take special care to be cognisant of this and respectful of the student's vulnerability. When done correctly, this can result in the establishment of a high level of trust in the teacher. Once established, this trust is a powerful motivator, but it is one-sided – the student is vulnerable, exposed, and trusting, while the teacher is not.

Alleged scandalous behaviour of a few prominent yogis has come to the forefront. These improprieties are nothing new, nor are they limited to yoga. Some have used their positions of power in inappropriate or even abusive ways. What becomes of those systems where the guru has been vilified and ousted? These revelations of "betrayal" have led to scrutiny of the whole of the discipline and calls to punish those who are perceived as transgressing. Despite the fervent acknowledgement of transgression, there is no clear path to forgiveness or plan for restitution or reconciliation. Where transgression has occurred, practitioners will decide if the system can survive the tarnished reputation of its creator or whether what they followed was the personification of the practice. Do they adhere to the system, or dispense with it for a less sullied course of study? This will continue to be a difficult challenge for yoga, as it has been in the past, and will require that scrutiny go beyond those implicated to the weaknesses in the culture of the industry itself.

Modern yoga has been critiqued as an elitist enterprise. Interventions have been proposed to rectify this unequal access; offering free classes and creating specialised programmes (e.g., Wounded Warriors, Black Yoga Collective, Full Body Yoga, Trans Queer Yoga, Justice and Equality Yoga) that provide a welcoming space for those who were once excluded. In addition to the desire to make yoga more accessible, these offerings "get people in the door". It may not initially be revenue producing, but it is a way to promote the studio (or the teacher) and does highlight the studio brand and what it stands for. Ultimately, studios aim to go beyond these discrete offerings and integrate diverse students into classes where the study of yoga becomes a shared enterprise. The challenge will be to overcome entrenched cultural divisions and develop a space where all are comfortable. This is, in part, a problem for the teacher for they must first acknowledge their own prejudices and then recognise that all students come to learn and be respected as individuals. Physical yoga is a malleable and resilient practice; therefore, teachers and participants need to examine in what ways its performance is an efficacious way to address social, political, and spiritual challenges. These are not necessarily outside yoga's remit, whether it involves any or all of these challenges. Physical yoga *should* promote intense and ongoing examination of the self, but this is a private and personal endeavour. A teacher can facilitate the self-discovery and self-regulation process of learning, but they cannot dictate it. For yoga to successfully accomplish accessibility, in light of the inequalities endemic in society, it will have to acknowledge these divisions and work to surmount them; focusing on the practice and addressing the following: (1) that yoga is subject to the same biases and beliefs found in society, (2) that injustices also existed throughout the history of yoga, (3) that it may be the teacher or the system of practice that is derelict when inappropriate discrimination occurs, and (4) that individual identity is fluid and nuanced, and specialised classes are a way to initially motivate involvement.

Since the time of Kapila and the pre-Socratics, the philosophic question of how to account for the obvious diversity in the world and still preserve the idea of unity has pertained. This conundrum is particularly relevant to contemporary yoga and its attempts to see cultural and societal difference as an unending process of respecting diversity *and* commonality. Will it be possible for teachers to pursue a philosophy that leads to a place of unchangingness or does one, through the practice of yoga, embrace the unceasing indeterminacy of reality? Those who prioritise experience over doctrine may have more success.

BORDERS AND BOUNDARIES

The yoga class and the act of teaching are negotiated experiences. The boundaries of this extemporised enactment are unspoken, but clear. Ideally, the teacher gives freely of their knowledge and the student accepts critical evaluation. The teacher has latitude to address anyone or everyone in the class and the student does not interfere with others' learning. The teacher establishes the models for achievement in the class while the student agrees to try wholeheartedly. The teacher sets the standards for decorum and the student adheres to these. Both the teacher and student avoid contaminating the classroom situation by leaving extraneous circumstances of their private lives elsewhere. The student does not draw undue attention to themselves – they ask only pertinent questions that the teacher accedes to answer. When the teacher does not know the answer to a question, they admit it and undertake research to find out the information or challenge the student to do so. If either teacher or student are shown to be wrong, they admit it and move on without rancour. In actuality, these ideal boundaries are subject to minor violations. Slight transgressions are glossed over because there is an understanding that dwelling on them impedes the learning process. However, there are occasions where this is not the case, and these lapses may lead to feelings of disillusionment or betrayal.

This disillusionment is sometimes the result of what happens outside of class. Disillusionment toward the teacher can be caused by a disjuncture in the way that the *role* of teacher has been portrayed and interpreted. The teacher who assumes the role of spiritually attuned vegan may believe in what they portray, but, if they are encountered by their students in a loud steakhouse bar (for whatever reason), they may expect there to be reactions that could range from delight to disappointment. If the teacher's characterisation in class is that of a paragon of purity, they set themselves a difficult standard to sustain. The situation is similar for the "maverick" – espousing iconoclasm gives students latitude to do the same in class, but this can be problematic when order and decorum are needed. Higher status professions come with the expectation that the personal and professional lives must match up, and, when they do not, disillusionment may result.

A teacher has authority and is therefore trusted by students in varying degrees. Their power is based on the garnering of social and cultural authority. A teacher that has both cultural and social authority will enjoy the highest respect. *Social authority* is granted by formal institutions in society and is vested in certification systems in contemporary yoga (whether these be by discipline or as recognised through a registering body like Yoga Alliance). This formal authority may also be acquired through "lineage" (either by birth or as a disciple), as the importance of one's teacher is a marker of status. *Cultural authority*, or influence, is gained through reputation. Unlike social authority, it is a measure of students' faith in a teacher and this evaluation is generally based on outcomes. A teacher without certification may enjoy immense popularity and high levels of cultural authority. A teacher with many certifications may lack cultural authority, and, therefore, the respect of students. Whereas social authority is relatively stable, cultural authority may be quickly lost or gained, but it is, in practical ways, more important. Teachers that have fallen from grace, for example, have lost their cultural authority, but not necessarily their social authority – without influence, their certifications, associations, and accomplishments fail to give them status or power. Maintaining cultural authority is paramount to successful teaching; without it, any number of certifications is useless.

Notes

1 See Geertz (1973) and Rosaldo (1973, 1980), as well as Boellstorff and Lindquist (2006), for a full and very interesting discussion of the relationship between emotion and culture.

2 Students who attend class with overtly oversized or round mats are often resented, as they are viewed as taking up too much space to the detriment of others.

3 There are some yoga studios that have a "mat-like" floor covering throughout the entire space, providing both acceptable levels of traction and cushioning, yet there are still students who find it preferable to use a mat; they feel more secure within the home space of the mat's territory.

4 Anthropologists recognise four basic kinds of political organisation: *Bands* and *Tribes* (which have a value of relative egalitarianism) and *Chiefdoms* and *States* (which are exemplified by increasingly hierarchical relationships). The selection of the term *Tribe* may reflect the value of egalitarianism in the yoga community.

5 Even if the Sun Salutations as we know them are a relatively recent invention, the practice of worshipping the sun in supplication has more primordial roots.

6 Inappropriate somatic dominance and other forms of abuse potentially arise from the power asymmetry inherent in the teacher/student relationship. There are a number of factors at play in each unique case of alleged abuse. Suffice to say that the teacher, because of their privileged position of authority, will be held responsible for these

infractions. Therefore, regardless of the circumstances, teachers should maintain clear boundaries between themselves and their students. When these boundaries exist, it becomes possible for the teacher to ask students to engage in the qualified risk necessary for yogic exploration.

Appendix 6: Reflection and Experimentation

The manipulations of status and role are ubiquitous in social interactions. People express dominance and submission in many ways; most notably by establishing territory and using both high and low status strategies to manipulate others. As a professional teacher, you establish and maintain proper boundaries with your students and colleagues as a way to keep the focus on the content of the yoga class. Creating boundaries and understanding the play of status allows you to better practice classroom management, express ideas with authority, and eliminate "drama" from your interactions. It is also an essential component in keeping your students and yourself safe from inappropriate relationships and interactions.

6.1 INAPPROPRIATE ADJUSTMENTS

Touch is full of cultural meaning and is a direct way to communicate information. The connotations of touch are changed when used for instruction in the form of adjustments. To be educational or explanatory, adjustments and assists need to be clear – ambiguity may lead to more everyday interpretations of touch. Physical corrections also risk injuring students, so they must be given with intelligence and care.

How would you describe an inappropriate adjustment? How would you respond to an inappropriate adjustment? How do you respond if a student believes you have given one? Are you confident that your adjustments are safe? How do you know if your adjustments are effective? What techniques do you use to ensure clarity in your physical corrections? How do you "read" whether the normal borders can be profitably crossed and how the recipient of your touch is left feeling when that border is re-established?

6.2 MODELLING BEHAVIOUR

Because of their higher status, teachers lead by example when they model appropriate behaviour. When hosting a guest teacher or attending another class, for instance, one thanks the teacher for adjustments and corrections. Through this ritualised formality, a teacher models how to create and maintain boundaries and show proper respect. A teacher presents themselves appropriately in dress, speech, and comportment, which models professional behaviour. A teacher prepares for class and models a dedicated work ethic for students.

What things do you consider when selecting yoga attire for teaching? Do you practice in front of your students? What kind of language do you feel is inappropriate for class instruction? How do you treat other yoga professionals; students from other studios or disciplines? Do you always come to class prepared or do you ask your students for suggestions? Is starting and finishing on time important to your students? How aware are you of the importance of your behaviour as a model for your students?

6.3 RECOGNISING BIAS

It is difficult, yet necessary, to recognise your own biases. Applying this awareness to your teaching can be even more challenging. Teachers are effective when they strive to treat everyone with the same respect even as they recognise individual differences. Avoidance does not constitute neutrality, nor does it mean you are treating everyone the same. The following questions entail self-reflection and the observation of personal behaviour.

Which "bodies" do you notice you avoid adjusting or correcting? What bodies are you more likely to pay attention to? What does this reveal about your inherent biases? How might you develop a curiosity about bodies – not just bodies of typical yogis, but all bodies? How might this help you treat all bodies with respect?

6.4 SCENARIOS – ARE YOU "STATUS FLEXIBLE?"

There are no "correct" answers to the scenarios below. Reactions in such circumstances are usually spontaneous and prescriptive solutions are difficult. However, familiarity with the possibilities for negotiating them leads to a better understanding and will aid in mitigating the results of impulsiveness. The aim is to lead back to the content of the yoga class and away from the volatility of social interactions.

How would a high-status teacher deal with the following situations? A low-status teacher? How would you manipulate status in reaction to these scenarios to ameliorate each situation?

- A group of students congregate their mats on one side of the room and are talking together just before class begins.
- A student rebuffs your corrections or instructions (high-status challenge).
- A student avoids your instructions by hiding in the corner or folding into Child's Pose (low-status challenge).
- The unofficial and unwelcome assistant teacher is giving instructions in class.
- Students are bothered by the noisy class next door.
- You are doing an outdoor class and a group of men walk by and start catcalling.
- A student monopolises your time just before class or just after.
- A student with a more advanced practice than you needs correction.
- An ambitious student is driven to achieve a posture, so they ignore your technical suggestions (e.g., kicking up into an inversion).
- Students are wearing inappropriate clothing that is too "revealing".

References

Ardrey, Robert. *The territorial imperative: a personal inquiry into the animal origins of property and nations.* London: Collins, 1966.

Boellstorff, T. and J. Lindquist. "Bodies of emotion: rethinking culture and emotion through Southeast Asia." *Ethnos*, vol. 69, no. 4 (August, 2006): 437–444.

Brown, Nina, Thomas McIlwraith, and Laura Tubelle de González. *Perspectives: an open introduction to cultural anthropology.* Arlington: American Anthropological Association, 2020.

Carissa, J., C. Cascio, David Moore, and Francis McGlone. "Social touch and human development." *Cognitive Neuroscience.* Accessed 14 August, 2020. doi: 10.1016/j.dcn.2018.04.009.

Ellingsen, D-M., S. Leknes, G. Løseth, J. Wessberg, and H. Olausson. "The neurobiology shaping affective touch: expectation, motivation, and meaning in the multisensory context." *Front Psychol.* vol. 6 (January, 2016) doi:10.3389/fpsyg.2015.01986. Originally published in print in 1986.

Geertz, Clifford. *The interpretation of cultures.* New York: Basic Books, 1973.

Gick, Judith. *The dangerous actor.* London: Virtual Angels Press, 1997.

Goffman, Erving. *Interaction ritual: essays in face-to-face behaviour.* London: Penguin Press, 1967.

Goffman, Erving. "The nature of deference and demeanor." *American Anthropologist* vol. 8, no. 3 (October, 2009):473–502. Accessed 5 October, 2020. doi: 10.1525/ aa.1956.58.3.02a00070.

Hall, Edward T. *The silent language.* New York: Anchor Books, 1973.

Johnstone, Keith. *Impro.* London: Faber and Faber Limited, 1979.

Levin, D.M., editor. *Language beyond postmodernism: saying and thinking in Gendilin's philosophy.* Evanston: Northwestern University Press, 1997.

Malbon, Benjamin. *Clubbing: dancing, ecstasy and vitality.* London: Routledge, 1999.

Morris, Desmond. *Manwatching.* London: Grafton Books, 1977.

Morrison, India, Line S. Löken, and Håkan Olausson, "The skin as social organ", *Experimental Brain Research* vol. 204 (2010): 305–314. https://doi.org/ 10.1007/s00221-009-2007-y.

Nevrin, Klaus. "Empowerment and using the body in modern postural yoga." In *Yoga in the modern world: contemporary perspectives*, edited by Mark Singleton and Jean Byrne, 119–139. London: Routledge, 2008.

Rosaldo, Michelle. "I have nothing to hide: the language of Ilongot oratory," *Language in Society* vol. 2, no. 2 (October, 1973): 193–223.

Rosaldo, Michelle. *Knowledge and passion: Ilongot notions of self and social life.* Cambridge: Cambridge University Press, 1980.

Somer, Robert. "Studies in personal space," *Sociometry* vol. 22, no. 3 (September, 1959): 247–260.

Chapter Seven
The Future of Practice

LOOKING TO THE PAST OR LOOKING FORWARD

Contemporary yoga looks over its shoulder to the canons of the ancients, while paradoxically involving itself in a whirlwind of syntheses of ideas and practices. Validity and authority are entangled with antiquity, leaving yogis to find circuitous routes to both argue and reinforce yoga's authenticity. In this context, will such a flurry of evolutions continue and what kind of link will they have with the past?

Contemporary fusions of yoga may have historical precedent, but the prolific rate at which they have been synthesised in modern times is a function of two things: the commodification of yoga and the perception that "plain" yoga needs to be made more "interesting". These interesting variations fall into two categories – those that mix the yoga with another somatic discipline (Yogalates, Yogabarre, Acroyoga) and those that attempt a fusion of the seemingly unlikely (goats and yoga, yoga and chocolate, yoga and beer). The commodification of yoga encourages the creation of new approaches (or new names) to boost attendance. Driven by market redundancy (many studios; many teachers of similar calibre teaching similar material), the entrepreneurially minded draw attention to their offerings by creating "the latest thing" and, sometimes, as with

DOI: 10.4324/9781003181910-8

Acroyoga, it shows staying power. It seems churlish to note the frivolous nature of some of these offerings. Kitten yoga – where kittens are allowed to cavort with practitioners in order to socialise with potential kitten adopters[1] has good intentions and a yogic rationale – "stress relief" – and very possibly is an amusing way to spend an hour. This is not to disparage "pop yoga" because it is not high-brow, it is delightful for what it is. In yoga, the "pop" question becomes one of degree – how much is a yoga class about the study of yoga itself and how much does the form of a yoga class serve to facilitate something else (whether it be fitness, stress relief, socialising, etc.)? "High-brow" yoga has a deserved place of importance; how will it carve out this place within the strictures of the commodified market?

Physical Skill and the Value of Experience

There is an expectation that the teacher should be exceptionally flexible and fit and have the greatest command of "tricky" postures. In the past, and in other somatic disciplines, teaching was not undertaken until one had reached, or was past, their peak performance. The teaching years commenced when individuals had sufficient experience and adequate command of a full and subtle range of skills. With the present emphasis on yoga as fitness, there is little need for a teacher to be experienced. Rather, the attractiveness of the teacher and some degree of ability fulfil the expectation of students and presumes that healthfulness and attractiveness can be equated. There is a sense that experience is valuable, but not that it takes years to accumulate. This is often why teachers now like to tell their inspirational stories as part of class – this is their level of "experience"; it is not wrought from years of practice – it is what brought them to or convinced them about yoga. In other somatic disciplines, like sport and dance, students will inevitably be "better" than their teachers as the somatic practice evolves. In yoga, there are more people doing extremely difficult postures than ever before. But, what remains unclear is just what exactly these extraordinary postures and practices are for. Athletes train so that they can compete; dancers do so in order to perform. But yogis do not utilise their physical skill set outside the practice setting. What uses will yoga be put to in the future, aside from the quotidian benefits it claims (stress reduction, fitness, sense of community)? Will the excellence that results from years of study be imparted to others who have similar discipline and the passion to carry forward the practice?

Because flexibility and impressive tricks have been valourised in yoga, people who have great backbends or can perform a handstand are considered "superior", even if they have limited knowledge and experience. This presumes that postural ability represents the highest level of achievement. The erroneous reasoning here is obvious; yet if the somatic practice is reduced to the performance of tricks or the recording of "cool postures" for marketing on Instagram, our understanding of deep yogic knowledge risks going in this direction.

The academic study of yoga has until recently been backward looking.[2] The historical view is certainly valuable, yet yoga, in its quest for authenticity, has been led to question its sources and explore innovative shapes and movements. Much like yoga, Modern Dance attempted a practical examination of its artistic motives. Its pioneers regarded the highly codified Classical Ballet as artistically stultifying. Though Modern Dance preserved some of the conventions of ballet, its search for artistic resonance led to the invention of new techniques, means of expression, and new "shapes and movements" on the stage. These shapes were without inherently specific meaning; the meaning was generated by the internal landscape of the performers and interpreted by the audience. As embodiment theory suggests, the body gives an indication of what is going on in the mind. In 1938, Martha Graham said that

> "Art is the evocation of man's inner nature. Through art, which finds its roots in man's unconscious – race memory – is the history and psyche of race brought into focus."
>
> (Brown, Mindlin and Woodford 1979, 50)

Though the language may appear out of date, the sentiment is clear. The inner nature (whether collective or individual) is what art, or yoga, evokes. It is not the postures or shapes themselves that have meaning; it is the qualities with which they are rendered. Physical yoga need not dispense with the canon of yoga systems (ancient or modern) nor need it be limited to these. Amongst its future aims may be the recognition that the spiritual landscape is revealed by the way practitioners execute postures. Yoga could build something new by embracing a plurality of styles and by cultivating what these different styles offer each other. The search for spiritual liberation is facilitated by technique – not everything is yoga. To quote Graham again, "If you have no form, after a certain length of time you become inarticulate. Your training only gives you freedom" (Mazo 1977, 157). Technique is the means through which physical yoga may display or communicate the spiritual landscape. The spiritual landscape is not about the external attractiveness of a person – it is something that is revealed through the way they enact what they do. Anyone, regardless of age, size, or social identity, with sufficient technical skill can render postures that reveal authenticity and spiritual validity. Ultimately, Modern Dance contributed to a revitalisation of ballet – new systems and priorities may do the same for the practice of yoga.

TEACHING YOGA IN THE FUTURE

The ease with which yoga teacher certification is acquired will result in two tiers of teachers – those who need certification to teach and those whose level of accomplishment has moved them beyond this requirement. The first group can conduct classes, and most will attract students who seek the sense of community that studios market. The second is a more niche group whose appeal is to students that wish to explore yoga more deeply as both a physical and philosophical pursuit. They may dispense with the idea of certification altogether because it is not necessary – their students attend for their knowledge (cultural authority), not their credentials (social authority). Those that prioritise community will attract students who like each other and who are, at least superficially, similar. Those that prioritise the deep study of self through yoga may have a more diverse clientele because the sharing of communal identity is secondary.

The future of yoga instruction does not lie in legislation by governing bodies, but in the constant exploration and renewed conception of basic themes and premises. These would include developing methods and techniques for practicing focus and concentration, refining and extending physical capacity, and the investigation of philosophic principles. Because cultural authority is important, students must be well informed consumers; they need to understand what constitutes good teaching and seek out excellent instruction if the quality of yoga teaching is to continue to improve. In a capitalist culture, where yoga is packaged and commodified, will this transpire? In many ways, consumerism encourages students to seek out the least expensive or most convenient class, despite the fact that they may know quality is lacking.

Since the 1970s, a major shift has occurred in the perceived tenets of yoga – a change from the seeking of an altered form of consciousness or experience of reality into a prioritising of "community".[3] With this has come a change from somatic procedures that intensely seek to alter or negate bodily/sensory engagement into the pursuit of an ethos of "non-judgemental" acceptance of who you are and a paradoxical concomitant notion that "transformation" can make you what you want to be. Conceivably, there could again be a movement towards a riskier exploration of consciousness through physical philosophy or even physical trial, requiring discipline, time, and dedication. However, the yoga industry today is a product of culture – its popularity results from a yearning for spiritual validation in a time when convenience is important, time is a luxury, quick fixes are desirable, and nurturing practices, like *yoga nidra* (yogic sleep), are in demand.

A non-judgemental ethos is intended to protect students from the evaluation of others and emphasise the democratic nature of the practice community. Through this perspective, all endeavours are deemed of equal worth; identified as uniquely perfect in their expression. In contrast, the practice of *critical acceptance* encourages students to listen to the insights of their teachers, determine what is useful in these critiques, and apply what is relevant for personal advancement. If the value of non-judgement is prioritised, approval becomes the only option (e.g., rounds of clapping for "giving it a go", respecting all executions as equal) and the process of learning is diminished, as the response is pro-forma. If opportunities for critique, especially those that are outside of the community's ethos, are not considered, the potential for these dissenting insights is lost. Criticism is a good thing if it is well informed, nuanced, and posits solutions. If, in the future, the community is the source of uncritical acceptance, this poses no less of a judgement than the critique of the teacher.

Courses and Classes

While teacher training courses provide a temporary relief for the financial dilemmas faced by studios running a weekly schedule of classes, there may be other solutions that are more beneficial to the studios, their students, and the quality of yoga teachers that trainings certify. Dance companies (and professional dance schools) sometimes have public classes, but often also have a course stream that is intended for aspiring professionals. Though public classes are available year-round, professional courses adhere to term times with breaks in-between to allow for the integration of students' learning and as a respite for trainers. Programmes vary from one, two, or three years depending upon participants' experience and require serious commitment and a prior level of accomplishment or at least aptitude. Prospective participants audition to get one of these coveted spots. Whatever their dreams might be, everyone acknowledges that a professional career will be difficult to attain; there are far fewer professionally realistic opportunities than there are candidates. Such realism is lacking from yoga teacher training in general. The teaching of yoga is the professional side of the industry and is a difficult career choice fraught with financial peril and considerable personal responsibility (and liability) for the welfare of those they teach. For those who want to intensively study yoga in a coherent programme, without the teaching component as a part of it, there are few options. Courses that address specific aspects of yoga other than teaching would be the most beneficial for the majority of students. Courses need not be as long, or as cohesive, as the model used to produce a dance professional. Initially, there might be short-term courses (e.g., twice per week for eight weeks) that would not commit the participants to something much more demanding than their present attendance. A course-based structure has business and educational advantages. Monies are taken upfront – the business knows how much revenue it has and can better budget its allocation. The student derives a sense of accomplishment that comes from completion. The teacher evolves a coherent structure for their subject matter and can set long-term goals for students in ways not possible in one-off classes. A course lays out a premise (e.g., working the breath in inversions) and then focusses on exploring the foundational material that supports it. It does not suppose that complete understanding or mastery can be obtained, but it gives enough information for continued study and appreciation of the foundation's relevance. The duration gives the participants time to digest and integrate what they learn. In this way, courses are different from workshops, which may attempt something similar but with a more compressed time for this integration.

Studios cite the reluctance of yoga students to sign up for courses as a reason for not implementing them. Somehow, a course is seen as too great a commitment to expect of the casual student. But, as an example, many of these same students have no problem signing up their children for a term of ballet or karate classes. Why is this the case? Possibly, they are willing to sacrifice spending money on their children but not themselves. They may believe their children can still learn and they themselves are too old. They may not value yoga as an educational enterprise and see it as "only exercise". Though yoga tights may cost more than a short course, tights are seen as a justifiable expense because they are a tangible item, whereas education has ephemeral value. People who conceive of themselves as "busy" see time as limited; committing to a long-term course may force them to miss out[4] on something else, and time or money spent on oneself seems indulgent, especially if one has nothing tangible to show for it. Though money spent on entertainment (concerts, cinema, restaurants, travel) is seen as worthwhile, yoga is perceived as lacking entertainment value and is a poor competitor against other amusements.

Without intellectual rigour, is yoga just playtime – not education and an inferior entertainment? Intellectual rigour, accompanied by physical form, can create a more entertaining class if the knowledge of the teacher is given an adequate forum to bring depth, development, and challenge to their teaching. A course format – multiple classes, thematically linked over an extended period, and attended by the same participants – would provide this. Courses, so conceived, are distinct from teacher training in that they are likely shorter in hours and more focused on an individual aspect of yoga. They require a smaller investment for the student and can be run continuously throughout the year. A business strategy would be to put the best teachers on a regular schedule of courses and to make these affordable. These courses would be the studio's investment in cultivating clientele for the more expensive teacher training enrollment. There is a place for classes that are meant to be one-off experiences; that are playful and undemanding, but this is only one option.

As teachers represent a pinnacle of understanding or accomplishment, teacher training should be the least common course and only open to those who are ready to do it. It is difficult to substantiate why a numerical value of 200 hours is the agreed standard for teacher training rather than the degree of accomplishment, but this has become institutionalised. In ideal circumstances, with participants who have strong practices and significant experience, 200 hours of work on pedagogical principles might be practical. Without substantial prerequisites for admission to teacher training, the broad topical demands mean that there is only time for a superficial coverage of teaching skills. Though teacher training is made to fit into compressed sessions (ten weekends or month-long retreats), it is rare for a studio to hold two or three per year. Scheduling is not the problem; rather it is because most studios populate their courses from their regular students, and it is difficult to sustain the turnover of new students to fill trainings. It is also short-sighted because every new teacher they create becomes a potential rival in the business of attracting new students. Teacher training sells the commodity of certification in the specialty of teaching and yoga courses sell education about an aspect of yoga. Studios may hold courses of varying lengths on a wide range of subjects that become prerequisites for their teacher training. This broadens the opportunities for students who wish to study yoga more deeply, and, for those who have an interest in teaching, it ensures a better foundation for training.

THE IMPACT OF TECHNOLOGY

Popular technology (such as *Fitbit*) provides easily accessible readings of calorific burn, heart rate, and oxygen levels during practice. Mats have been designed with built in sensors to record and respond to foot placement and weight dispersal, accompanied by set classes that give interactive instruction – providing real-time feedback within a few basic parameters and promoted as a way to get individually tailored corrections. While these are modest technological innovations, there are others that pose interesting possibilities for experiencing yoga. There are a number of ways that body sensors and wearable motion capture devices could be employed to make the experience of yoga both highly creative and relevant to self-education. In 1920, Louis Theremin invented a musical instrument that is played by a performer moving their hands between two antennae connected to oscillators. This made it possible for movement to create music. In 1984, composer Edward Williams refined this idea in a project that sought to enable dancers to create and shape the music that accompanies them with their own body movements (Soundbeam, 2020). He designed an ultrasonic movement-to-MIDI converter that enabled electronic instruments to be played from a distance by body movements in an ultrasonic beam (Wikipedia, 2020). The resulting tech-nology – *Soundbeam* – uses ultrasonic sensors to detect movement and translates this into sound. It has found practical use in music education and in the aged care sectors and could be adapted to yoga movement.

Motion capture, which is also referred to as motion tracking, is the method of recording movements of people and objects. Motion capture systems work by making use of one or more sensors (AZoSensors 2014)[5] worn on the body. If the body sensors' information is set to a music soft-ware program, the information can be translated into musical sound or control lighting levels. For example, the movement of the wrist through space can be the sound of a violin, or the rotation of a joint could control the level of intensity or colour of a light. One could use one's body to compose music or make the studio space like a light show. If *vinyasa* is practiced with evenness of breath and evenness of movement, the use of such technology could measure to what degree this is true. If this is equated with evenness of mind, it may be imagined that the spirit as well is visually or aurally illustrated with such measurements. This has the potential to change the experience of yoga – through gestural/postural-musical interface, a class might engage in making music together and self-practice could be similar to composing music. One could have the immediate feedback of light or sound to monitor the way in which they perform their yoga.

YOGA AS ART

Art places its subject in a context – it puts a frame around it. It does not endeavour to tell the whole story of reality, but to imply underlying truths. Physical yoga should be an excellent subject for the arts – it inherently contains themes of balance and harmony as well as mystical ecstasy and the struggle with failure and spiritual discontent; and, of course, the transitory nature of life and reality. Yet, physical yoga, both as art and a subject of art, is rarely created within the studio or elsewhere. In the visual arts, photography has been the most successful – resulting in coffee table books of collected and commissioned photos and occasional gallery exhibits. Though yoga as a sculptural subject has not attracted many artists, it may have a considerable future – it certainly has a rich past. The postural nature of yoga makes it ideal subject matter – one where the model is actually "in the pose". Marc Quinn's sculptures of Kate Moss (the actual posture was modelled anonymously) – Sphinx (2006, cast in bronze) and Siren (2008, cast in gold) – shows the figure in a posture with both legs wrapped behind her head. It is intricate and slightly lurid – somehow capturing both the difficulty of yoga and a contemporary sexuality mingled with celebrity – apposite for this era. Filmmaking is another discipline (documentary and fiction) that explores yogic themes and has attempted to apply yogic premises to modern sensibilities. Films like *The Matrix*, *Bagger Vance*, *Groundhog Day*, and *Star Wars* have reinterpreted ancient philosophical tenets (the universality of the search for meaning and immortal nature), though without overt use of physical yoga.

As a vocabulary for the performing arts, physical yoga has had influence on Indian dance forms as well as Modern Dance and ballet. Outside of the studio, physical yoga is occasionally performed in short exhibitions of technique at yoga conferences, festivals, or even shopping malls. Sometimes set to music, these are usually the performers' "greatest hits" – a series of difficult postures strung together as a complex sequence that might occur in a very advanced class. "The class" is the context and the work done in class is the usual range of the performers' expressiveness. Groups such as *DeRose Art Company* (Brazil) and *Tripsichore Yoga Theatre* (London) have successfully ventured into the theatrical realm and show that there is considerable scope for performance that is yoga based in the future.

Confining Yoga in the Virtuous

The focus on the inspirational in contemporary yoga has erased much of its imagery in the popular imagination. This is not to descry the worthiness of material that is uplifting, but, as seen in the Smithsonian Institution's Arthur M. Sackler Gallery exhibit *Yoga: The Art of Transformation*, historically, the art of yoga has been far more intentionally disturbing and complex in its representations. As Michael O'Sullivan states in a review of one portrait, "She's [Bhairavi] wild-eyed and red-skinned, wearing a necklace of human skulls. Her lap also is full of them, and she's sitting, in the lotus position, on a headless human corpse, one of several dismembered bodies scattered about the landscape, through which cadaver-eating jackals roam" (O'Sullivan 2013). The exhibition showed that the art of yoga was a powerful subject and deserving of a place for serious consideration in a gallery or museum setting. Likewise, it revealed the intensity with which yoga was practiced and the high stakes it entailed. As graphically described by Cotter Holland:

> Some of these images are pure escapist fantasy, with handsome yogi princes devoutly tracking down sweethearts in Sufi romances. Other pictures have the specificity of photo-documents, as in the case of an extraordinary double-leaf 16th-century painting of a mortal fight between rival yogic sects. The skirmish, waged over bathing rights in a sacred river, was witnessed by the Mughal emperor Akbar, who described it to an artist, who in turn spares us none of the bloody details of yogi-on-yogi stabbings, spearings and decapitations ... What's great about the Sackler show, apart from the pleasures of its

images, is that it not only lets us see the history of that practice in action, but understand how radical it was.

(Holland 2014)

The exhibit and accompanying catalogue contain many portrayals of yoga practice and practitioners that "contradict the contemporary stereotype of yoga" (O'Sullivan 2013). The material is daring and frightful. Much of it would not be condoned within the comparatively anodyne world of contemporary yoga, with its ethos of "acceptance", which leaves out the possibility that "The All" also contains the wrathful, the frightful, and the horrific.[6] There is a censure of nearly anything that does not evoke "positivity"; the struggle in yoga is not often depicted. Failure, confusion, and frustration are rarely a part of the artistic discourse of contemporary yoga; instead, a "peaceful" or "ethereal" frame surrounds most artistic representations.

Yoga Photography

Photography of yoga stands apart from the other arts, because, in seeking to capture a moment of stillness, it approximates the efforts of a yogi in a posture. The success of the "art" of yoga photography has been partly driven by its prosaic uses for marketing. It successfully bridges the worlds of art and commercialism. Though video is also used, the still image is particularly apt for conveying the postural nature of most physical yoga. Photographs sell workshops, even when their descriptions are indifferently worded.

Yoga photography often uses quixotic juxtapositions – headstands in the street; balances on precarious rocks; black and white studio shots with atmospheric light and shade – which convey something quite different (and are meant to) from the actual yoga studio experience. Some are extraordinarily beautiful and demonstrate the superb technical skills of the photographer and model. They certainly have quality and may find a lasting place as artefacts. But will that be because of what they reflect about the spiritual endeavours of yoga? Apart from their compositional clarity, will they speak across the ages? Increasingly, this is dependent upon the digital revolution. As long as photographs can be sourced digitally, they will survive, but if they have no physical counterpart in the world, they may be lost. Coffee table books, calendars, or yoga themed collections of photos for galleries may have greater longevity. *Instagram* and *Facebook* are predicated on the rapid recording and sharing of images but place less emphasis on their artistic or lasting value. The future may see photographs curated in different ways – exclusive online access, gallery sections of websites, and monitors with slide shows in yoga studio reception areas.

When so many people have a camera at their fingertips and shots can be doctored digitally, good photographs abound. Great photographers, however, have both technical mastery and an ability to recognise and sympathetically capture their subject in situ. While a photographer like Henri Cartier-Bresson was renowned for being in the right place at the right time, it is difficult to capture decisive moments in a yoga studio. A photographer snapping shots is an unusual occurrence and, while observed, people are less likely to behave candidly. Furthermore, the conditions can be problematic – lighting is often unsympathetic, studios are cluttered with props, gym bags, and scattered clothing, and people are placed randomly throughout the space. The mat, with its rectangular shape and block of colour, often clashes with the organic human form. The increasing ubiquity of the camera and the commonplace nature of self-documentation, along with the ability to edit the extraneous from images digitally, may mean that everyone could get better at creatively evoking the yoga experience within an idealised studio context.

Yoga Music

Music is popular because it adds ambiance and context to a class. The modern yoga teacher often takes on the role of DJ and some share their playlists online. However, little music has been written and recorded that is specific to physical yoga practice – rather it is generic and could accompany many activities. The relationship of music to yoga movement (or any movement) is implicit, ambiguous, and extensive as well as having profound physiological effects (such as tears or shivers) (Sloboda 1991, 110). While it may be obvious that music touches our sentiments and brings on bodily responses, Suzanne Langer suggests that it also can call forth "emotions and moods we have not felt, passions we did not know before" (Langer 1942, 222). Music intimates the ineffable to us. As Iain McGilchrist puts it in his summary of Schopenhauer's thought on the subject, music "is highly particular, and yet seems to speak of things that are universal" (McGilchrist 2009, 77). This will certainly remain an important aspect of how the teacher uses music in the future.

The use of recorded music in classes is not free unless you have permission of the copyright owner, which may subsist (depending on where you do it) in a number of ways – with the composers, the publishers, and the recording itself. As it constitutes a public performance in many countries, there may also be licensing arrangements that need to be made just to play music before an "audience" of students. There are organisations that provide fully licensed music for such uses as yoga classes, and it is likely that more of these will develop in the future. While the range of music on offer from these organisations is vast, much of it is stylistically generic and, though it may serve as yoga *muzak* (background music), it is rarely intended for specific use – it is up to the teacher to fit the class to what is on offer if the music is to play a role other than setting the mood.

Live music is another matter. Accompaniment for movement is a particular skill. The musician either musically describes what they see, interprets what they sense from the movement, or leads the character of the movement to be expressed. When it is skilfully done, there is a reciprocity. In an era when yoga is sensitive to cultural appropriation, it is curious that many teachers feel they are espousing authenticity by playing instruments like the harmonium (invented in France in 1840) to accompany their classes.[7] Kirtan "call and response" is rarely used in physical practices but is a ready staple of class playlists. Kirtan's rise in popularity parallels that of yoga and has seen some kirtan bands make use of instruments and musical arrangements that are not traditional. Musicians who have knowledge of rock or pop music have incorporated these elements and created "pop Bhakti". This trend is likely to continue as teachers seek musical accompaniment for their classes that appeals to their clientele as "authentic".

A preoccupation of contemporary yoga has been with "how to take it into the world". Yoga art is one solution to this. It is distinguished from the practice itself, but, in the case of physical yoga, it takes the skill set of practitioners and, through creation, gives expression that validates the spirit and its limitless capacity. The more it deliberately veers in the direction of "art", the more ambivalent it is likely to be in its meaning and function. Its ambiguity is its strength because it invites interpretation.

ONLINE TEACHING

The business of yoga was thrown into turmoil in 2020 with the coronavirus pandemic. The closure of physical premises and the movement to online "spaces" brought unforeseen problems to the fore. The context of the teacher was altered – some presented themselves in their bedrooms/ living rooms and some chose a "virtual" background. Those with actual studios used these somewhat eerily empty spaces.

The online medium is better adapted to the headshot – to accommodate the full body longshot, eccentric camera angles abound. When teachers address students in a studio, it is rare for the teacher to speak so directly – face to face – as they are compelled to do at the beginning of an online class. Teachers' conventional rituals for beginning classes are replaced with the informalities of "admitting" students and subsequent "muting" of audio. In the demonstration of material, the teacher needs to decide whether or not to face the camera (where it is easier to monitor their own image and, to some degree, the students) or to turn 90 degrees to be side on; possibly giving a clearer idea of the profile of the shapes they make but losing some of the contact with the camera and students. Visually inessential space frames their demonstration. In a studio class, the student dismisses this from their visual field. The sonic problems of instructing while playing music become hard to reconcile, as it is difficult to objectively monitor the relative levels of voice and music while teaching, and music and image are often asynchronous.

Online teaching may prove reasonably effective; whether interactive or pre-recorded. However, even in interactive online teaching, where there are opportunities for the teacher to observe and instruct in real time, the actual experience of communication is diminished. This is more so for the teacher than the student (whose attention is experiential and about self-discovery). The aural and visual cues that let a teacher assess their effectiveness are less easily accessed – the practicalities of needing to mute the audio of the participants mean that the sound of breath is lost for the teacher and the monitoring of multiple students on a small screen mean that much subtlety is lost visually; particularly because of the difficulty in assessing three-dimensional forms in a two-dimensional format. Buffering speeds of the video can also cause problems. None of this is insurmountable, but it does mean that the teacher has to process layers of reality that do not exist in live classes. This is mitigated by the delight of having people from remote parts of the globe take part in the same experience. Faster buffering, more adaptable cameras that pan and zoom and that can be teacher controlled, and improved sound that allows for multiple sources are developments that would be welcome.

Pre-recorded classes provide an opportunity for the teacher to concentrate on the format of class and production values without the distraction of students; much like DVDs and videos have in the past. They may also be edited to create clarity for students or provide different angles to visuals. What the teacher gains in production value and polish, they give up in responsiveness to students. However, recorded and online classes are convenient; one can do yoga any time one wants and with nearly any teacher, stopping and starting as one pleases. But something is lost when the "specialness" of time and place is sacrificed. One of the delights of teaching is seeing a student "get" something. Absent a responsive audience, the teacher may find it difficult to enjoy teaching and students may also miss the direct engagement with the teacher.

The movement to online spaces also opens intriguing possibilities. Recorded and edited classes have more scope for multiple cameras and shot selection as well as post-production refinement for sound. Increased online content offers students greater opportunity for research and recorded short segments of technique, for example, can deal with specific technical issues that students can research online. Students' work on individual portions of a class can be filmed outside of class time and submitted to the teacher for private review; they can spend more time framing their questions and the teacher is able to give a more measured and personalised response. Recording offers the teacher greater opportunity to review their classes and better evaluate the effectiveness of their teaching. Recordings give a reference for the student – they can see themselves as the teacher does and better understand corrections. Recording sessions for private clients offers an added opportunity to give useful reference materials for their continued home practice.

Some features of online teaching are likely to show further divergence from in-person instruction. Corrections are more general and, because the teacher's main point of reference is their own body, they will be more often generated by what they notice in their own practice than by what comes from the students. Online private classes are less problematic; the teacher can devote all their attention to the one or two students they are instructing, giving real-time feedback. Both the lack of teacher scrutiny and the distractions of a home environment force students to be more personally responsible; without a teacher present, students are free to put less effort into work or opt-out altogether.

Yoga is a potent somatic discipline because it demands risk. Though advertised as "safe", advancement, as in any discipline, demands a level of challenge. The skilled teacher is always on a tightrope with regard to the demands they make of a student – what they assess to be physically and mentally appropriate. Online, there is less scrutiny, and the teacher has limited information on which to base their assessments. Therefore, the teacher may resist challenging students (whose safety they cannot ensure). With fewer demands and diminished scrutiny, online instruction becomes less risky and, at the same time, potentially more dangerous. The lack of oversight, ironically, may also afford some teachers a level of freedom as they can teach what they like, without the constraints of attunement to individual students. This may lead to increased progress for students who might not otherwise be exposed to such challenges in studio classes.

What remote instruction always lacks is the ability to give physical adjustments and assists. To compensate, teachers may give an abundance of verbal cues. This can be cumbersome when there are many students needing different cues, or if the instruction is for a moving sequence. In any event, words do not function in the same direct experiential way as touch; they are simply suggestive. Another option is for students to be given instructions for self-adjustment. To do this, they are brought into a tactile relationship with something other than themselves (wall, floor, block, chair, etc.). In online classes, students use mundane objects, improvising with what is at hand. This encourages the student to see what a prop "does" and if and when they are necessary. In place of the teacher's touch, students can give themselves self-adjustments through techniques like binding and the use of mudras. In this case, the student uses themselves as the "other" in the self-adjustment process.

LEGACY: ARTEFACTS AND MONUMENTS

A culture's rubbish can become an artefact for present-day investigators. For archaeologists, this leads to insights about the mundane and the cosmological concerns of the people who wrought them. What will the future make of yogic artefacts and what might be generated by this era of yogis that could be monumental? Will a selection of surviving Instagram posts – like Harrapan seal equivalents – reveal the concerns of the present day? How might a future archaeologist interpret the ruins of a yoga studio in North America where they discover a statue of Shiva and a long since discarded yoga mat with designs derived from art thousands of miles away?

An artefact refers to any humanly manufactured article that now has cultural or historic interest. Under the rubric of yoga, an extraordinary amount of material meant for public consumption is generated daily: *Facebook* and *Instagram* posts, newsletter blogs, podcasts, and website promotions. Peer review becomes reduced to numbers of "followers" and "likes" and subject to astute marketing strategies and algorithms. There appears to be little concern for what might make a long-lasting contribution to yoga and its practices. Are social media posts the apotheosis of yoga ambition and how might the materials that appear in social media be made to assume a more long-lasting form?

The disposability of contemporary yoga artefacts, like mats and calendars and social media, is a powerful philosophic statement. In previous eras, artworks such as statuary, paintings, and drawings were used as stimulus for meditation. Contemporary yoga artefacts are mostly quotidian – their uses are principally mundane and so is the interpretation of them. A mat is for practice – when it wears out, it is disposed of unceremoniously; photographs are for marketing, although they may have secondarily been appreciated for their artistic value; calendars are beautifully designed but are meant as practical record keeping. The interpretation of such objects is in their usefulness. The studio altar is crowded with a mix of artefacts that are both mundane and sacred – pictures of teachers, books, singing bowls, statuary, incense, candles, and posters of chakras. These are mostly mass-produced commodities but are potential artefacts, as these mundane items will determine how today's yoga will be interpreted in the future.

Other aspects of yoga culture may survive into the future. Styles of physical practice based on unchanging series of postures may have staying power. Their codified nature detailed in books, posters, and recordings, as well as the potential for a continued living practice, may ensure this. Will there be any Gorakhnaths, Marichis, or even Shankacharyas? Today, celebrity is short lived. The multiple lineages derived from Krishnamacharya may make him a candidate for long-lasting fame. Some yoga literature may survive – published research has a breadth of scope and a pragmatism that ensure it endures. Books that are chiefly pictorial may have lasting appeal because there is a timeless artistry to the photography and the models' execution of the postures. Conferences and festivals are currently social gatherings or opportunities to take a class with a famous teacher rather than places where research is debated and shared. They have not functioned to effectively advance yoga as a serious discipline but may do so in the future.

The Monumental

Monuments are of a different order – they are meant to last – they imply a different conception of time. There was once an assumption in archaeology that the transition from the Mesolithic to the Neolithic – from nomadic hunting and gathering into stable settlements – came about because of the development of agriculture; reasoning that people had to remain in one place to tend to the land and livestock and that this gave rise to the creation of monuments. However, the creation of monuments in the landscape appears to have preceded agriculture. In northern Europe, "the first monuments may be found *alongside* the first domesticates, and sometimes the earliest evidence for more intensive land use does not come until *after* mounds or cairns had been built...what they find instead of houses are monuments...[and they] seem to have played a specialised role in a landscape in which other signs of human activity are dispersed and often ephemeral" (Bradley 1998, 10). Such monuments are interpreted as mortuary and point to a ritual perception of time and space that differs from the every day. Not only did they provide a mnemonic and symbol for the past and the dead, but their existence was also of a permanence that long outlived their creators.

Monuments are built to last and inspire a perception of the past living in the present as well as a projection of their future duration. A substantial physical edifice provides the living with a tangible means to structure relationships with dead ancestors and to those yet to be born. Therefore, the actions that people perform in temples or stone circles are often done in prescribed rites, which have a marked consistency and are unlike the more improvised nature of actions performed in day-to-day living. The video screen of online yoga has become like a monument. It is a curious situation where the student is often in the "normal" home environment of their bedroom or living room, where they turn their attention to a video screen to observe the teacher in a far-off location and begin to do the kind of physically repetitive movements and rhythmic breathing required by a yoga class – doing overtly prescriptive actions that mark ritual rather than the mundanely performative. This is not exactly the same as veneration, but it does share features of it – the highly focused attention, actions performed in rhythmic fashion that are without obvious mundane utility, and a sense of space where one can, in a sense, inhabit another world (for the student this is the teacher's studio or room). The internet could be construed as a monumental and devotional object and it encompasses an idea of a space that spans the globe where beliefs and memories are stored.

Though online teaching may share some aspects associated with the monumental without wholly satisfying the notion of a physical edifice that is long lasting, it is still likely to provide a legacy. There may be ideological reasons why contemporary yoga has yet to create the equivalent of temples hewn from stone and decorated with statuary of *gurus* and acolytes in yogic postures. In the introduction to *Yoga: The Art of Transformation*, Tamara I. Sears observes that such statuary depicts "a dramatic ontological shift at the level of the soul. Because knowledge of yoga gave the practitioner the potential to transcend the realm of human existence and enter a state akin to becoming divine, it was restricted to highly accomplished *gurus* and their most dedicated pupils" (Sears 2013, 47). Though, in the past, such statuary may have celebrated the achievement of mastery by the individual *guru*, the ethos of contemporary yoga celebrates the greater plurality where the self is already "perfect" and does not need to gain such prowess. Nor does it require the creation of a monumental edifice to sustain itself.

The search for one's own power is an individual endeavour. The creation of a monument requires enormous, concerted group effort and an envisioning of what it will become. The yoga community shares beliefs based in the values of freedom and individuality, promoting self-love, self-acceptance, and self-development. These individually focused efforts do not require ineffable ideas about reality or monuments to extoll them; they require no symbology or metaphor to grasp. If a monument is to be created, it will require concerted action aside from the promotion of self-advancement. It needs to identify and stake claim to a "territory". The monument of yoga this generation bequeaths may not be a physical one, but rather a legacy of lasting respect for theory and practice.

CONCLUSIONS

Modern yoga is practiced internationally in many variant forms and fusions. Some of these practices retain aspects of yoga's surmised aboriginal past, and some require a stretch of the imagination to see why they would be called "yoga" at all. At the heart of any traditional practice of yoga is the quest for some kind of knowledge; knowledge that leads to a greater understanding of self and of the nature of the universe. Which of the many competing perspectives (e.g., fitness, therapy, self-love, self-improvement, immortality, spirituality, etc.) will gain ascendancy in a world that valourises individualism, and how will these ideas be passed down from teacher to student?

Philosophy or Religion

Today, there is much debate about whether yoga is a philosophy or a religion. Positive psychologist Marcello Spinella believes this debate to be a purely modern conundrum, for, at the time of the inception of Eastern traditions like yoga and Vipassana meditation, there was no distinction between science, religion, or philosophy.[8] Religion was the "science" of pre-scientific thought; it was the discipline through which universal phenomena were explained. Later attempts to naturalise "religious" explanations – to speak of "nature" as explicable and demonstrable – were radical in that they forced a shift in disciplinary modalities. Meditation and yoga, Spinella believes, were more akin to incipient systems of psychology. They explained the working of the human mind in the context of universal experiences of living. These systems attempted also to explain experientially why human beings were "imperfect" when compared to the divine, and, at the same time, why humans were unique compared to other lifeforms. Although this distinction was moot in the past, today it stands at the centre of much debate about yoga as a discipline; should it be regulated or not, can one practice it alongside another religion without dissonance, is it practiced for supernatural ends either in this or the next life? Or is yoga simply a way to better understand and participate in the lived human experience? And might all this really depend on how one defines philosophy or religion in the end? How the yoga community defines itself whether in a singular or multiplicity of ways will determine how it evolves in the future. The more important question, therefore, for the individual yogi and yoga as a discipline is what impact the designation of "philosophy", "religion", or even "science" will have on yoga's evolution.

Preconception Versus Objectivity

As a yoga practitioner, one measures each experience against what one thinks they already know. Theories developed in the past comprise this kind of preconceived knowledge; they inform, but at the same time they threaten to limit one's ability to notice things that are not expected to be there. A practitioner might mitigate this bias by approaching each experience as if it were novel, suspending preconceptions. One can equate this to the field method of *participant observation* (in anthropology) where research questions are discovered and developed through the experience of observation itself.[9] This method allows the yogi, embedded in the experience of practice, to come to conclusions that are less influenced by their assumptions.[10] This is not to say that one can ever be free of bias or the knowledge gained from previous experience. It is a way, however, to detach oneself from dependence on philosophical analyses of the past, and our current beliefs, long enough to evaluate their efficacy. Analysis of the past, using textual or prehistoric sources, is always marked by a degree of speculation. Since there is no living witness to the practices of the past, a reliance on the primacy of textual analysis in understanding yoga philosophy and practice is not immune to this speculation. There is merit in looking to the past, however. It allows the researcher to consider the history of ideas and how knowledge is generated, and it often produces insights into modern philosophy and practice. But, if yoga is to be a living practice, it cannot rely so heavily on these texts as a way to structure personal beliefs, nor as a definitive source on the nature of human experience. As a practitioner, one is the only vehicle for that experience and the meaning found within it. Yoga, like anthropology, is less an "experimental science in search of law" than it is "an interpretive one in search of meaning" (Geertz 1973, 3–32).

Magical/Scientific Thinking

The practice of contemporary yoga is often coupled with radical or even magical thinking. The ability to imagine another reality is quite useful when engaging in creative exploration or when one attempts to discover new truths. But what happens when this is accompanied by a denial of demonstrable facts like scientific data – when trust in entire disciplines, rather than particular beliefs, is abandoned? *Hatha* yoga texts make references to various alchemical and magical transformational powers of postures, breathing, or meditation practices, as does the third chapter of the *Yoga Sutras*[11] and the questioning of these ideas, which are obviously spurious, may be discouraged in contemporary yoga since questioning threatens the legitimacy of the system as a whole. If Peacock

Pose does not make us immune to snake bites, as yogic lore suggests, and headstands fail to make the hair turn black again (Aiyar 1914, 124(b)–125), or opening our hips fails to release negative emotions, then what of the other claims that yoga makes? With increased knowledge comes the abandonment of ideas that, though once embraced, are now seen as erroneous. For some, this new knowledge may be countered with the entrenchment of specious beliefs; for when systems require dogmatic adherence, they become rigid and unable to adapt to change. When one uncritically accepts the claims of the ancients as real – without ever having witnessed them – and design experiences around them, one loses the important objectivity needed to engage in experimentation. They engage in magical thinking, instead of critical thinking.

Chapter 5 examined how a disregard for empirical information can lead to the questioning of facts and the rejection of modern scientific knowledge. This can make one susceptible to the manipulations of false *gurus*, snake oil salesmen, pyramid schemes, and unfounded conspiracy theories because it presupposes that *the modern* cannot be trusted. This likely creates a high degree of cognitive dissonance,[12] which can have profound and lasting psychological impact on practitioners. In a culture of "nonjudgement", will the yoga community be capable of sufficiently critiquing its own tenets and practices? The practice of *critical acceptance* provides a starting point for creating a solid foundation upon which such introspection might happen. Through critique, especially self-critique, a discipline is made more robust and ideas may be exchanged in service of its evolution. But, when occultism and elitism intersect, and knowledge is understood as secret and only available to the chosen (as is stated in the ancient *hatha* yoga texts)[13], the opportunity for scrutiny of any kind is threatened.

Ethnocentrism and Modernism

In addition to rejecting modernism and science, and their concomitant institutions, yogis often valourise indigenous or aboriginal practices as untarnished "true" knowledge. Various disconnected practices (sweatlodges, ayahuasca, rebirthing, shamanic rituals, etc.) are incongruously combined into what is imagined as an unbroken tradition of superior and interrelated folk wisdom. This wisdom, viewed as changeless and pristine, is believed to be suppressed or ignored by the supposed evils of modernism. In anthropology, this is known as the ethnocentric belief in the *noble savage*, one who is untarnished by civilisation and at the same time superior to it. But all cultures gain knowledge over time – cultures change and grow – they invent new ideas through innovation and borrow ideas from other cultures through the process of *diffusion*.[14] The members of any culture (like their practices) are not museum relics frozen in time. They are living beings with agency, curiosity, and aspirations. To believe otherwise bespeaks of a certain arrogance, one that is in search of ancient wisdom, which, in fact, is as modern as our own. What will become of yoga if magical thinking displaces scientific reasoning, and indigenous knowledge and various energetic principles are conflated (Bender 2010)? The lack of rigour with which yoga practitioners currently accept and integrate beliefs and practices into their own threatens to weaken the integrity of the discipline. It is up to modern practitioners to behave as *participant observers* as they do experiential/experimental research and test the results through introspective means.

The study of the self and the scrupulous identification of that which is not essential, but merely the accretions of one's nurture and nature, might ultimately lead to this understanding: that whatever it is that constitutes "I" – consciousness – is something inherent in all things. This premise suggests an essentiality that is the foundation of a "wholeness made up of diverse forms" and that, by studying the self, one can gain understanding of that which, in appearance, is not the same as the individual. In seeking to understand the ineffable reality of all that is other than self, a focus on self-validation lacking the ongoing process of critical, tentative, and innovative exploration runs the risk of self-deception or over-simplification. One may seek to satisfy the hunger for self-validation through participation in communities, examination of past methods of training and theory, as well as modern science and health practices. However, the social sphere (communities) is an uncertain phenomenon of reality; research on the past is subject to contemporary bias, and science and health practices are only tools to aid this search and not ends in themselves. Because of the changing nature of reality, we are challenged by uncertainty; systems of science, philosophy, religion, and yoga are our attempts to hold this at bay, but such propositions are impermanent solutions – they are destined to be altered by revelations of one kind or another. When new systems of practice or models for yoga community evolve in the future, they too will be altered either by upheaval or erosion. Inexorable change will move things on. Like all things in *prakriti*, its organisation or codification – the material coming into being – is the beginning of its end. The strength of "the spirit" – of consciousness – is its ability to imagine; to embrace potentiality (*purusha*) – to take from "that which is possible" and to facilitate its creation. It takes a measure of responsibility for that which is created – the spirit may be imagined as an artist whose palette and canvas is reality.

In and Out

As David Loy has stated, "Whether you shrink to nothing or expand to incorporate everything, it amounts to the same thing: there's no longer the sense of separation between inner and outer, between me and the world" (Loy 2012). The general position stated in Chapter 1 was that *asana* presented a technical approach to finding an irreducible self by looking inward and that *vinyasa* sought a state of profound understanding by looking outwards. Various systems of physical practice are extolled in modern yoga and they fall somewhere in a spectrum between these two polarities. Systematising yoga (whether it be as codified series of postures, or by construing yoga as community practice, or as a healthful pursuit) is part of a necessary, yet ultimately provisional, attempt to control that which is unpredictable. Analysing or proving a system's or community's efficacy through statistical evaluation, or measurement of tissue elasticity, or sociological implications are highly creative efforts that change little about reality itself. To provide insight into reality, the information and details they provide still must be assembled into a cohesive form that accounts for the diversity and commonality of phenomena. This is the paradox that yoga confronts – for all the uncertainties and inevitable unpleasantness in reality, there is also a "delight" – a bliss of entering into the crazily unpredictable lucid-dream world of reality and a mocking of its apparent control over our lives, which can only end in death. Yoga posits that, upon the death of a person, the "I" of consciousness carries on in others – its potentiality does not cease. Each act contributes to this reality and its effects reverberate onwards in ways that are uncertain and unpredictable, but always fascinating.

Notes

1   See Laneri (2018) and BBC (2018) for examples.
2   See Jain (2015), Wildcroft (2018a), Bender (2010).
3   Wildcroft's (2014) dissertation illustrates one example of the many intentional communities at the centre of modern yoga. These communities are often formed

around common interest, studio membership, or lifestyle choices. Identity in these communities is often defined in opposition to hegemonic institutional structures like "lineage", "biomedicine", "toxicity", or "capitalism".

4 FOMO (fear of missing out) is a modern cultural phenomenon.

5 Including photosensors, angle sensors, IR sensors (infrared sensors detect radiant heat), optical sensors (measure the quantity of light), accelerometers (sense motion and velocity), inertial sensors (measure acceleration and velocity along three perpendicular axes), and magnetic bearing sensors.

6 See White (2011) for depictions of sinister yogis.

7 Rabindranath Tagore called the harmonium the "bane of Indian music" and also said "As the player finds all these notes ready for use, he needs only a little deftness to play it, and the result is a torture only fully appreciated by those who have undergone it." Rahaim (2011, 657).

8 Marcello Spinella, P.C. 29 November, 2020.

9 In participant observation, the anthropologist enters the field without a research question and by living, participating in, and observing the culture being studied over an extended period of time, forms a research question and a frame of analysis as it is revealed. This requires that one be as objective as possible.

10 "The greatest enemy of good ethnography is the preconceived notion" (McCurdy 2006, 4). But preconceptions are also the enemy of the yogi or any "objective" observer.

11 *Yoga Sutras of Patangali*, Vibhuti Pada III: Union Achieved and Its Results (any translation), describes powers ranging from knowing all knowledge, time travel, invisibility, walking through objects, and having the strength of an elephant, among many others.

12 Cognitive dissonance is the state of having inconsistent thoughts, beliefs, or attitudes, especially as relating to behavioral decisions and attitude change.

13 *Siva Samhita*, 1.19, *Hatha Yoga Pradipika* 1.11 (any translations).

14 The movement of an idea, practice, or product from one culture to another, albeit in an altered state, which allows it to more easily fit into the receiving culture's existing worldview.

15 Ashtanga Yoga (Jois) defines certain "injuries" positively, as "openings" (Donahaye 2019).

Appendix 7: Reflection and Experimentation

7.1 THE PROBLEM OF PRECONCEPTION

As one accumulates knowledge, they inevitably form preconceptions on which they base their interpretations of experiences. While this information is critical to creating meaning, it also threatens to limit the objective analysis of these same experiences. For instance, if you have been taught to associate the sensation of pain in your hips with the release of "emotional trauma" (or an "opening")[15], this association between physical and emotional release will tend to be both accepted and confirmed. This may be the case even when one is physically injuring themselves in this effort (rather than emotionally healing). How might you encourage students to enter new experiences suspending preconceptions? How do you do this in your own practice? What do you imagine will be the greatest challenges to objectivity as yoga evolves (e.g., lineage, philosophical beliefs, conceptions of health and wellness, social identity)?

7.2 THE FUTURE OF LINEAGE

Theodora Wildcroft's (2018b) study on post-lineage yoga describes a movement away from lineal affiliation and the authority that these lineages hold. What lineage(s) do you see yourself allied with? What aspects of these do you think should be preserved for future generations? What might be dispensed with? Is the role of the yogi to rebel against tradition or to uphold it?

7.3 YOGA EXHIBITIONS

The popularity of physical yoga has resulted in many people pursuing extreme postures requiring unusual flexibility, strength, and balance. While acquiring these attributes is undoubtedly personally rewarding, can such skills be applied in ways that have particular utility beyond the studio? Dancers, acrobats, and contortionists practice similar skills of balance and flexibility so that they can be used expressively in performance.

There is a tradition of giving yoga exhibitions. What is the scope for taking yoga into a public setting? Does the idea of performing or watching yoga at a shopping mall (the beach, the theatre, a nightclub, a church, etc.) seem offensive? If so, why? Do you feel the same if you see or hear a youth choir performing in a similar space? What are the differences? What are new and practical uses for the skill sets of physical yoga?

7.4 YOGA ETHICS: INTENTIONS AND RESULTS

How might yoga be a force for good in the future? How important is engagement in the world versus self-development? Is a disciplined or dedicated (regular) practice intrinsically virtuous? If so, how does that work? Why is (isn't) it an exercise in vanity? Is the intention behind a regular practice more important than the result? Will doing yoga with good intentions make you an ethical person? Are good intentions enough to ensure that yoga will evolve as a discipline? How do you distinguish your intentions from your actions and their results?

7.5 THE FUTURE OF TEACHING ONLINE

Most students report that the online experience has more distractions than in-person classes. The lack of physical corrections and assistance further distances the student from the teacher. The difficulty of carrying out a dialogue with questions and answers may leave students' queries unanswered. To accommodate this, teachers may find it necessary to institute before and after sessions of informal question and answer. How does one creatively overcome the problems posed in online teaching?

What are the merits of classes recorded and made available at any time versus the special occasion? How much does the lack of a facility and props for practice affect teaching? How might this be resolved (strategies, props that are improvised, or nonstandard yoga props)? Ideally, how will yoga accommodate new technologies for teaching in the future?

7.6 IF YOU WIN THE LOTTERY

If you win the lottery and can invest unlimited funds in a Yoga Institute, where would you locate it? Who would teach there? What sort of structure and physical features would it have? What curriculum? Does the yoga you teach and your vision for it change when you have an ideal space?

References

Aiyar, K. Narayanasvami, translator. *Yogatattva Upanishad of Krishna-Yajurveda*. Madhu Khanna, editor of original publication. Madras: Tantra Foundation, 1914. Accessed through PDF. www.purna-yoga.ru/en/library/text/ancent/Yoga-Tattva_Upanishad.pdf.

AZoSensors. "Using sensors to capture body movement." 11 September, 2014. Accessed 3 September, 2020. www.azosensors.com/article.aspx?ArticleID=429.

BBC. "Kitten yoga: the class where you can play with feline friends." Broadcast 22 July, 2018. www.bbc.co.uk/news/av/world-44915459/kitten-yoga-the-class-where-you-can-play-with-feline-friends.

Bender, Courtney. *The new metaphysicals: spirituality and the American religious imagination*. Chicago: University of Chicago Press, 2010.

Bradley, Richard. *The significance of monuments*. London: Routledge, 1998.

Brown, J., N. Mindlin and C. Woodford, editors. *The vision of modern dance: in the words of its creators*. Princeton: Princeton Book Company, 1979.

Donahaye, Guy. "Ahimsa? Practice with Pattabhi Jois – pain and injury." 1 January, 2019. New York: Ashtanga Yoga Shala. Accessed 4 December, 2020. www.ashtangayoga.nyc/pattabhi-jois/2019/8/14/ahimsa-practice-with-pattabhi-jois-pain-and-injury.

Geertz, Clifford. "Thick description: towards and interpretive theory of culture," *The interpretation of cultures: selected essays*. New York: Basic Books, 1973, 3–32.

Holland, Cotter. "Eons before the yoga mat became trendy." *New York Times*, 2 January, 2014. https://www.nytimes.com/2014/01/03/arts/design/yoga-the-art-of-transformation-at-sackler-gallery.html. Accessed 14 June 2020.

Jain, Andrea R. *Selling yoga: from counterculture to pop culture*. Oxford: Oxford University Press, 2015.

Laneri, Raquel. "Screw cat yoga — kitten yoga is here, and it's adorable." *NY Post*, 17 April, 2018. https://nypost.com/2018/04/17/screw-cat-yoga-kitten-yoga-is-here-and-its-adorable/. Accessed 14 June 2020.

Langer, Suzanne. *Philosophy in a new key: study in the symbolism of reason, rite and art*. Boston: Harvard Paperbacks, 1942.

Loy, D. "What is non-duality?" Talk given at Spirit Rock Meditation Center. *Awakening in service and action: a study retreat on socially engaged Buddhism*, 25 May, 2012.

Mazo, Joseph H. *Prime movers: the makers of modern dance in America*. New York: Morrow 1977, 157.

McCurdy, David W. "Using anthropology," In *Conformity and conflict*, 12th Edition, edited by J. Spradley and D. McCurdy, 422–435. San Francisco: Pearson, 2006.

McGilchrist, Iain. *The master and his emissary: the divided brain and the making of the Western world*. New Haven: Yale University Press, 2009.

O'Sullivan, Michael. "'Yoga: the art of transformation' art review." *Washington Post*. 31 October, 2013. www.washingtonpost.com/goingoutguide/museums/yoga-the-art-of-transformation-art-review/2013/10/31/774039c0-3da9-11e3-a94f-b58017bfee6c_story.html.

Rahaim, Matt. "The ban(e) of Indian music: hearing politics in the harmonium," *The Journal of Asian Studies*, vol. 70, no. 3 (August, 2011): 657–682.

Sears, Tamara I. "From guru to god: yogic prowess and places of practice in early-medieval India," *Yoga: the art of transformation* (catalogue) at the Arthur M. Sackler Gallery, Washington: Smithsonian Institution, 2013, 47–57.

Sloboda, John A. 1991 "Music structure and emotional response: some empirical findings," *Psychology of Music* vol. 19, no. 2 (October, 1991): 110–120. https://doi.org/10.1177/0305735691192002.

Soundbeam. "History." Accessed 3 September, 2020. www.soundbeam.co.uk/history.

White, David Gordon. *Sinister yogis*. Chicago: University of Chicago Press, 2011.

Wikipedia. "Edward Williams, composer." Accessed 3 September, 2020. https:// en.wikipedia.org/wiki/Edward_Williams_(composer).

Wildcroft, Theodora. "Patterns of authority and practice relationships in post-lineage yoga" PhD thesis, London: The Open University, 2018a.

Wildcroft, Theodora. "Post-lineage yoga." Blog post yoga and thought from Theo Wildcroft, 20 April, 2018b. www.wildyoga.co.uk/ 2018/04/post-lineage-yoga/.

INDEX